Contents

Part 1: The Basics **1**

Questions 1-6 give background information about breast cancer with such topics as:

- What is cancer?
- Will I die if I get breast cancer? Is it true that breast cancer is the leading cause of cancer death among women?
- What causes breast cancer? How do I determine whether I'm at risk?

Part 2: Risk Factors and Prevention **15**

Questions 7-22 discuss risk factors and ways of minimizing breast cancer risk:

- What risk factors are most important in determining my likelihood of getting cancer?
- My breasts are always lumpy. Does this mean I have cancer or that I'm at a higher risk of getting cancer?
- How does estrogen relate to breast cancer? Can birth control pills or hormone replacement therapy put me at risk?
- I've heard a lot of different theories about what causes breast cancer. How do I tell which factors should concern me? Should I do research?
- Is there anything I can do to prevent breast cancer?
- What is a breast self-examination (BSE), and why should I perform one? When should I start doing BSEs? How often should I do BSEs?

Part 3 Diagnosis **49**

Questions 23-26 outline the steps in determining whether you have breast cancer:

- I've found a lump in my breast. What should I do now?
- How is a mammogram performed? Is it uncomfortable? Does it hurt?
- What might show up on a mammogram and what results should concern me?

Part 4: Treatment   65

Questions 27-56 give an extended overview of treatment options, treatment side effects and complications, options for breast reconstruction, and prospects of recurrence:

- What should I do if it turns out I *do* have cancer?
- What are the options available for the treatment of breast cancer?
- What is a mastectomy and how does it differ from a lumpectomy? Why would I choose one over the other?
- What is radiation therapy?
- What is chemotherapy? How is hormonal therapy different?
- What is meant by adjuvant therapy? Is it the same as alternative therapy?

Part 5: Coping with Treatment and Side Effects   153

Questions 57-68 address issues related to pain, hair loss, and other side effects. Practical matters such as financial and legal issues related to treatment are also discussed:

- How can I relieve the pain associated with treatment?
- What happens if the dose of pain medication I get isn't enough? Are pain drugs addictive?
- What can I do to deal with hair loss?
- Do meditation and guided imaging really help prevent recurrences?
- I can't afford the medicine for chemotherapy; can I use half the dose? Where can I find help with the expense if I don't have insurance?

Part 6: Changes Cancer Brings   177

Questions 69-84 discuss ways to cope with emotional and physical changes that occur after cancer diagnosis and treatment:

- How do I get my life back to normal?
- Is it normal not to have mood swings when diagnosed, or will there be a delay in that response?
- What role does past pain, anger, stress, and fear play in this disease?
- My body seems different now that I have cancer—I don't feel as attractive. What can I do to change this?
- Why is it so difficult to tell friends and loved ones about my cancer diagnosis?

Foreword

In the fight against cancer, knowledge is power. So when Zora Brown and Harold Freeman asked me to contribute to the second edition of *100 Questions & Answers About Breast Cancer*, I was absolutely delighted. Both of these individuals are pillars of the cancer community. I have known Zora Brown through her groundbreaking work as a vocal advocate for all people facing cancer, and Harold Freeman's service as a volunteer leader of the American Cancer Society has been immensely valuable to our organization's progress against the disease. Both bring unrivaled experience to this book—Zora as a courageous survivor and Harold as a passionate crusader for reducing the cancer burden among the medically underserved and one of the country's most influential advocates for increasing access to medical care for diverse populations. Perhaps most importantly, they bring a genuine passion for improving the lives of every person touched by breast cancer and a deep commitment to someday seeing it eliminated altogether.

To previous generations, cancer was a mysterious specter—a disease few understood and even fewer survived. Now, thanks to advanced knowledge about prevention, earlier detection through screening, and innovative new therapies, more people than ever before are surviving. In fact, breast cancer death rates in the United States have decreased steadily for more than a decade, and they continue to decline. Survival for localized breast cancers now stands at an inspirational 98%. Even cancers that have spread regionally are 80% survivable. I sincerely believe the ultimate defeat of breast cancer is a dream we can—and certainly will—achieve.

Until that time though, no one is immune to cancer. It spares no community, age group, or family. And when a personal cancer diagnosis comes, it is a shock and a clear threat to all those things we hold dearest—health, time, and life itself.

In November 2004 we learned that my wife Carole had breast cancer. Thankfully, it was detected at the earliest possible time. She has completed her surgery and radiation beautifully—facing cancer with her usual positive and upbeat attitude. Indeed, her courage has been an inspiration to me.

When Carole was diagnosed, I more fully came to understand what cancer survivors and their loved ones experience when they hear those dreaded words. It surely must be one of life's most vulnerable moments. And yet, comprehensive public awareness efforts—including books like this one, written by dedicated, informed professionals—have helped transform cancer from a hopeless disease into one of the most preventable and curable of all life-threatening diseases.

This book will help you face every aspect of the journey ahead. Zora Brown and Harold Freeman know that a breast cancer diagnosis prompts scores of questions—and that they don't always occur to you when you're in the doctor's office. This book will allow you to get comprehensive answers to your most pressing questions from a source you can trust. In addition to helping you work through your physical and emotional concerns, I hope this book will bolster your courage and strength and inspire you to persevere.

The message I hope you will take from this book is simply this: You are not alone. Take comfort in the support of your loved ones and friends. They will continue to be the light that guides you toward recovery. Reach out to others who share your breast cancer experience. Find courage in each other's strength and hope in each other's friendship.

Breast cancer is undeniably difficult, but it does not define you. You remain the same wonderful and unique person you were before your diagnosis. Never lose faith in yourself and your capacity to endure. Treasure your many blessings, and learn from each day of this journey; ultimately, it will make you even stronger.

John R. Seffrin, PhD
CEO, American Cancer Society

Preface

In recent years, breast cancer has become widely recognized as a critical issue in American health care. With new diagnoses numbering in the hundreds of thousands each year, raising awareness among women of the need to monitor their breasts for signs of disease has proven effective in lowering the death rate for this cancer. Information on how to screen for, prevent, diagnose, and treat breast cancer has been rapidly developed and disseminated to the general public—perhaps too rapidly. A recent article in *The New York Times* noted that the multitude of new studies and recommendations (which sometimes contradict one another) create confusion and uncertainty in the general public as to how to proceed. The recent controversy over mammography is a case in point: we are told by one group of scientists that women 40 and over should have yearly mammograms, but others say that mammograms are ineffectual before age 50. Many experts—including the authors of this book—still support the use of screening mammography for women in their 40s, but when the opposite opinion is emphasized in the media, whom should the average woman believe? A newspaper article reports promising new treatments being tested at a prominent university hospital, but there's no indication as to whether approval is imminent; how do readers learn more? We see on television that the FDA has approved several new drugs for use in breast cancer; how do we find out about them, and how do we determine which one is best? In the age of the Internet, a Web search of the term "breast cancer" will bring up hundreds, if not thousands, of Web sites with topics ranging from scientific studies of the molecular biology of cancer, to inspirational stories about cancer survivors, to rumors, myths, and wild exaggerations about the causes of breast cancer. How does anyone—particularly a person who never thought about cancer before and hoped she'd never have to—make sense of all this?

In *100 Questions & Answers About Breast Cancer*, we bring different perspectives on cancer to a collaboration that we hope will assist newly diagnosed patients in navigating the mass of confusing, often conflicting, information available to them. **Zora Brown**, founder and chairperson of Cancer Awareness Program Services (CAPS) and the Breast Cancer Resource Committee (BCRC), is a 20-year breast cancer survivor who has worked for many years to promote breast cancer prevention, awareness, and education for women, particularly women of color. Brown has received numerous awards and honors, including the 2001 Spelman College Community Service Award, the 2001 Avon National Community Advocate Award, the 2001 Coalition of 100 Black Women, the Women of Valor Award, and most recently, the United Negro College Fund's 2002 Measure of a Person Award. She is an outspoken advocate for minority and women's health issues. **Harold Freeman,** MD, is the founder and Medical Director of the Ralph Lauren Center for Cancer Care and Prevention. He is currently a Senior Advisor to the Director of the National Cancer Institute (NCI). He holds the academic rank of Professor of Clinical Surgery at Columbia University College of Physicians and Surgeons. Dr. Freeman is one of the foremost international authorities on the interrelationships among poverty, culture social injustice and cancer and is the leading voice on cancer disparities. **Elizabeth Platt**, an editor and science writer for Jones and Bartlett Publishers, Inc., is the daughter of a breast cancer survivor and an editor of journals and books on cancer. Aware of her own increased risk for the disease, she discovered just how difficult it could be to navigate the ever-changing landscape of cancer information when looking for details on cancer risk factors and prevention strategies.

The information in this book is a synthesis of current medical standards, advice based on our experience, and good, old-fashioned, practical common sense. We wrote this book to help newly diagnosed patients make sense of the diagnosis and learn some of the things you can expect will happen. Above all, we want readers to understand that as a cancer patient, you don't have to be a cancer *victim*; you can and should ask questions, request help when you need it, and participate actively in making decisions about your treatment. We could not cover all topics as thoroughly as we would like, nor could we answer every question that's out there, but we've tried to present the best information available on many important topics while pointing our readers in the direction of high-quality sources of information and encouraging them to ask questions and seek assistance. We hope that our efforts will help some of the many women (and their families) who will confront breast cancer in the months and years to come.

Many people assisted us in writing this book. We would like to thank Chris Davis, Executive Publisher, Medicine at Jones and Bartlett Publishers, Inc., for approaching us with the concept. We thank Susan Troyan, MD, FACS, for reviewing the manuscript and suggesting updates. Zora Brown thanks her mother, Helen Brown, who taught her to ask questions and to seek solutions; her husband, Kenneth Rowland, who gives her the inspiration and support to be able to follow her passion; her familial sisters, Joyce, Belva, and Margaret; her community of sister survivors; and her niece Monica Botts, whose probing quest for answers to her heritage led to the development of many of the questions. Special thanks to Zora's "buddies." Elizabeth Platt thanks her mother, the Reverend Nancy Van Dyke Platt, for guidance, encouragement, feedback, and a top-notch example of how to survive cancer; Pat Morrissey, Shellie Newell, and Tovah Lazaroff for their encouragement and offers to read over the manuscript; Gail Wilkes for her careful proofreading and comments; and special thanks to Mark, Thomas, and Marcayla for patiently tolerating the many weekends that Elizabeth couldn't come out to play.

DEDICATION

I dedicate this book to my beloved sisters Belva Brown Brissett (1941–1990) and Margaret Brown Brady (1947–2002). I do so with immense gratitude and hope.

Though they both lost the battle against breast cancer, they instructed me, by the examples of their own lives, not how to die, but how to live. Their courage in the face of adversity, their spiritual strength in the face of mortal weakness, their capacity for giving, and their hope in the face of hopelessness, shall abide with me forever.

But for the generosity of their spirits, their spirituality, and grace, and dignity, the Breast Cancer Resource Committee would not exist; I could not have endured; my great resolve to fight breast cancer on every front might have been weakened, and this book would not have been written. Thus, I dedicate to Belva and Margaret much that I am and all that I hope to be.

Zora Brown
2006

Risk, Action, and Hope in the Battle Against Breast Cancer

Zora K. Brown

This book is born of experience: not just my experience with breast cancer, but my family's, and the experiences of my sister survivors. For me, breast cancer was a journey that began before I was born. Both my great-grandmother and grandmother were diagnosed with breast cancer at a time when little was known of this disease—and there was little reason for hope. Mammography had not yet been invented; genetic factors were unknown; radical mastectomy was virtually the only treatment option; and the survival statistics were grim. No one knew what caused breast cancer, so it was something to discuss in whispers—a secret shame. Its presence was concealed behind euphemisms: "The Big C" or "Woman's Disease," or just "IT." So powerful was the stigma of cancer that women like my great-grandmother and grandmother kept silent about it; so little did they anticipate recovery that they merely resigned themselves to inevitable death, with only their faith in God to sustain them.

It is often said that the Lord helps those who help themselves. In many ways, for those willing to seek answers, help has arrived in the form of knowledge. We have many more resources to fight breast cancer than we did in the time of my great-grandmother, because we know so much more about the disease. We know now, for instance, why cancer has struck five generations of women in my family, the Brown family from Oklahoma: a genetic defect handed down from mother to daughter that predisposes us to breast and ovarian cancer. We also know that, as African–Americans, the women of the Brown family and others like us are at risk for more aggressive cancers that strike earlier and have higher fatality rates. Medical advances in mammography, surgical techniques, genetic screening, chemotherapy, and hormonal therapy have enabled us to watch for signs of cancer, to catch its appearance earlier, to treat the tumors before they spread, and even to accomplish something unthinkable to earlier generations: **cure it**.

But this book is not exclusively about medicine. It's also about hope. It's about finding the will and strength to fight for your life in the face of a disease that is still dreaded by women everywhere, but is no longer a shameful secret. It's about holding your head high in the face of a silent enemy. It's about fighting cancer with weapons beyond medicine—with hope, humor, spirit, and positive thinking. These are weapons I got from my mother—weapons that my sisters and I have used to our own and others' benefit. The third generation of Brown women confronted with cancer was the turning point: my mother, also diagnosed with breast cancer, faced the same limitations as the women who preceded her, but she found the strength to overcome them. She used her knowledge of family history and emerging medical advances to fight back; she resisted the impulse to resign herself to death by cancer. Her hope, optimism, and desire for information to aid her fight were passed on to her four daughters. These strengths proved critical as, one by one, each one of us was diagnosed with cancer. Three of us—and later, my brother's daughter—were diagnosed with breast cancer before the age of 35; each faced recurrences; my sisters, Belva and Margaret, and my niece all have died. I was diagnosed with breast cancer at 32, and subsequently underwent two separate mastectomies.

Understanding my family and racial histories taught me to be alert; years before my diagnosis, I began to take precautions such as regular self-breast examinations and mammograms, a macrobiotic diet, the identification of excellent physicians, and the best medical insurance possible. Although this knowledge did not render me immune from breast cancer, it did facilitate its early detection, which helped me survive when it did strike—and has kept me alive for the nearly 21 years since my initial diagnosis. As has been so aptly documented, family/genetic history is but one among several high-risk factors. In reality, to be a woman is to be at risk of breast cancer. One in eight women will get breast cancer in her lifetime, regardless of family history; for families like mine with genetic pre-dispositions, the risk is extraordinarily high. But as a member of a high-risk family, my sisters and I, and now our nieces, have come to understand that we have been given, not a genetic curse, but a gift—the gift of knowledge and the inspiration to use that knowl-edge to address the challenges of breast cancer, and to imbue other survivors with hope.

And hope there is, in plenty. In the last decade alone, breast cancer research, prevention diagnosis, and treatment generally have greatly advanced our war against its ravages. High-risk families now have at their disposal a number of potential options unimag-ined by my ancestors, or even by myself and my peers. Free pre-screening tests for high-risk patients are available to anyone. Early detection methods such as regular self-breast examinations and rou-tine mammography are widely promoted. Breast cancer prevention studies are becoming inclusive of all races and income brackets. Isolation of the BRCA1 and BRCA2 genes and the use of promis-ing new drugs hold enormous promise in preventing cancer in high-risk patients. All of these factors add up to one thing: *Breast cancer is a disease you can survive, even if you're at high risk.*

This book is based upon the premise that survival proceeds from knowledge—not knowledge that frightens or inhibits, but knowledge that inspires us to take responsibility for our own sur-vival into our own hands, that galvanizes us into action on our own behalf, that vanquishes despair and ignites hope. Such sentiments gave rise to the Breast Cancer Resource Committee, a nonprofit organization that my late sister Belva and I founded to promote education and resources, particularly for African-American women. Since its inception, the Committee has conducted over 1000 breast cancer awareness and education programs nationwide. These initiatives include media promotions; securing grants to sup-port mammography screening for low-income women; initiatives to encourage early diagnosis and treatment; provision of prosthesis and surgical garments to low-income women; peer counseling and support groups; testimony before Congress, Federal, and local government agencies on breast cancer issues; and, of course, initiatives aimed particularly at high-risk family members.

PART ONE

The Basics

What is cancer?

Will I die if I get breast cancer?

What causes breast cancer?

More ...

1. What is cancer?

Every organ in the body is made up of various kinds of **cells**, which are easily distinguished from one another in form and function. Brain cells are different from blood cells, which are distinguishable from liver or skin cells, for example. Cells normally divide in an orderly way to produce more cells only when they are needed. Each cell is preprogrammed to have a specific life cycle, and normal cells contain a trigger that begins the process of cell death. This process of regulated growth and death helps keep the body healthy.

Occasionally, cells become abnormal and divide without control or order, or fail to die at the appropriate time. If cells divide when new cells are not needed, they form too much tissue. The mass or lump of extra tissue, called a **tumor**, can be **benign** or **malignant**.

Benign tumors are not cancer. They can usually be removed, and in most cases, they don't come back. Most important, the cells in benign tumors do not invade other tissues and do not spread to other parts of the body. Benign breast tumors are not a threat to life.

Malignant tumors are cancer. The cancer cells grow and divide out of control; they also become **undifferentiated**, which means they lose the distinguishing characteristics of the original tissue. They can invade and damage nearby tissues and organs. Also, cancer cells can break away from a malignant tumor and enter the bloodstream or **lymphatic system**. That is how breast cancer spreads and forms secondary tumors in other parts of the body. The spread of cancer is called **metastasis**.

The Basics

Cells

basic elements of tissues; the appearance and composition of individual cells are unique to the tissue they compose.

Tumor

mass or lump of extra tissue.

Benign

not cancerous.

Malignant

cancerous; growing rapidly and out of control.

Undifferentiated

cells that lose the distinguishing characteristics of original tissue.

Lymphatic system

a collection of vessels with the principal functions of transporting digested fat from the intestine to the bloodstream, removing and destroying toxins from tissues, and resisting the spread of disease throughout the body.

Metastasis

the spread of cancer.

Carcinomas

cancers that form in the surface cells of different tissues.

Epithelial

cells on the surface of a tissue.

Sarcomas

cancers that form in connective tissues.

Many women survive for years after being diagnosed with breast cancer.

Cancers in general come in two forms: **carcinomas**, which form in the surface (or **epithelial**) cells of different tissues, and **sarcomas**, which form in connective tissues. Breast cancers are carcinomas.

2. Will I die if I get breast cancer? Is it true that breast cancer is the leading cause of cancer death among women?

Breast cancer is a very frightening and dangerous disease, but it doesn't necessarily mean you will die if you get it; many women survive for years after being diagnosed with breast cancer, and a significant number are cured completely. How any individual case turns out depends largely on how far the cancer has progressed and what the woman and her doctor do to treat it.

There is a lot of good news when it comes to breast cancer. First, death rates from breast cancer are on the decline. Second, if caught early through self-exams or mammography, breast cancer can be cured. Third, advances in detection and treatment continue to improve **prognosis** and provide hope even to women with advanced cancer or with a genetic predisposition to breast cancer. Some of these advances are discussed later in the text.

Prognosis

an estimation of the likely outcome of an illness based upon the patient's current status and the available treatments.

According to the American Cancer Society, lung cancer, not breast cancer, is the leading cause of cancer death among American women; however, breast cancer is a close second, and when you consider only women between the ages of 40 to 55, it comes in first. The fact is, the only reason breast cancer isn't the principal cause of cancer death among women of all age groups is because it is much easier to screen for, detect, and cure than lung cancer. Breast cancer is the most common form of cancer in women in the United States, with over two million breast cancer survivors currently living in the United States today. The National Cancer Institute estimates that roughly 182,000 new cases of breast cancer were diagnosed in 2001.

3. What causes breast cancer? How do I determine whether I'm at risk?

If you are a woman, you're at risk for breast cancer—but your chances of getting it may be low, moderate, or high, depending on a number of **risk factors**, which are discussed in later sections. The fact is, no one factor can be pinpointed as the cause of breast cancer, but a complicated combination of many considerations can increase the chances that a woman will get it. Statistics from the National Cancer Institute's Surveillance, Epidemiology, and End Results Program (SEER) publication *SEER Cancer Statistics Review 1973–1997* show that an average woman's lifetime chance of getting breast cancer are 1 in 8.

Risk factors

any factors that contribute to an increased possibility of getting cancer.

DID YOU KNOW that you don't have to be female to get breast cancer? A small number (less than 1%) of breast cancers diagnosed in the United States occur in *men*. In 2001, approximately 1500 men were diagnosed with breast cancer in the United States; approximately 400 men die from the disease each year. Many of the risk factors for women (age, weight, heredity, and hormonal activity) appear to be the same for men; likewise, the symptoms that tell a man or his doctor that there's a problem tend to be similar. As with breast cancer in women, early detection is a key ingredient to successful treatment, but because men generally aren't screened as women are, often their disease goes undetected until a more advanced stage. A man showing symptoms similar to those discussed for women—breast lumps, discharge from the nipples, a sudden change in the appearance of his breasts, and so forth—should talk to his doctor about checking for breast cancer. If you have concerns or questions about male breast cancer, refer to the appendix for Web sites and resources.

So, how do you know if you're likely to be the "one" who gets breast cancer? A woman's risk of getting breast cancer is composed of a number of factors. The good news is, some of these factors can be controlled—diet, weight, the level and frequency of exercise, and use of alcohol are all elements that influence a woman's risk of breast cancer, and all of these can be changed (though some are changed more easily than others). The bad news is, some factors are either beyond a woman's control or are difficult to control: these include general attributes, such as race and family history of cancer, as well as attributes specific to the individual, such as a history of diseases such as uterine and ovarian cancer, as well as overall physical history. Physical history includes a woman's current age, the age at which she had her first period, whether or not she had children, whether or not she breast-fed a child, how old she was when she had children, or the age at which she reaches menopause. The important thing to understand is, while you can do nothing about many of the factors affecting your risk level, just knowing where you stand with respect to any or all of them can help you determine how concerned—and how vigilant—you need to be.

The National Cancer Institute offers an online risk assessment tool that can help you quickly and easily ascertain your risk level. See Question 15 for details on how to locate this service.

4. Does breast cancer only affect breast tissue? Are there different types of breast cancer?

The term "breast cancer" describes a whole group of concerns that begin in the breast and can sometimes spread outside of the breast. It is important to note that breast tissue is not limited to what most women think of as their breasts, but is found above, below, and to the side as well. That's why, when performing a self-exam (see Question 13), women should take care to feel the areas underneath their breasts, in their armpits, and above the breast as well. Cancer that **metastasizes,** or spreads to other organs, is the same disease and has the same name as the primary (original) cancer. When breast cancer spreads, it is called metastatic breast cancer, even though the secondary tumor is in another organ. Doctors sometimes call this "distant" disease. Metastatic cancer of any sort can damage the organs it invades. The earliest metastasis usually occurs in the **lymph nodes,** which is why diagnosis and treatment of cancer targets not only the affected breast, but the lymph nodes in and around the breast as well (see Questions 25, 31, and 36).

There are two structures in the breast where cancer strikes most commonly. The breast is divided into approximately 20 **lobes,** which somewhat resemble bunches of grapes; the individual "grapes" are called **lobules,** and the "stems" of the bunches are called **ducts.** Lobules produce milk, and ducts carry the milk from the lobes to the nipple during breastfeeding. Cancer beginning in the lining of the ducts, called **ductal carcinoma,** is by far the most common form of breast cancer. Cancer can also form in the lobules; this is referred to as **lobular carcinoma.** Though it is much less common, it is more likely to occur in both breasts or in separate locations within a single breast. There are other, rare types of cancers, such as inflammatory breast cancer and Paget's disease, which begin in the breast as well. These will be discussed in more detail further on.

The Basics

Metastasize

cancer that spreads to other organs.

Lymph nodes

tissues in the lymphatic system that filter lymph fluid and help the immune system fight disease.

Lobes

collections of lobules within the breast.

Lobules

individual glands within the lobes that secrete milk.

Ducts

the passages within the breast that bring milk from the lobules to the nipple.

Ductal carcinoma

cancer beginning in the lining of the ducts.

Lobular carcinoma

cancer formed in the lobules.

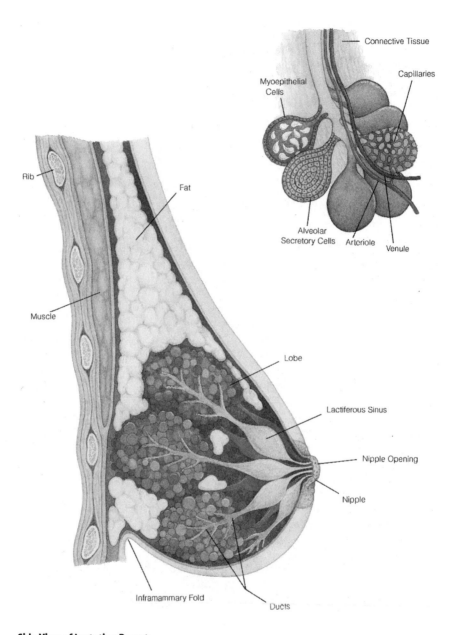

Side View of Lactating Breast

5. What are the different types of breast cancer? What is the difference between invasive and noninvasive cancers?

The single most important factor in assessing any breast cancer is determining whether it is noninvasive (in situ) or invasive. This will determine your treatment path and, to some extent, your expectations for results.

Noninvasive or **in situ** cancers confine themselves to the ducts or lobules and do not spread to the surrounding areas. There are two main types of noninvasive cancer: **ductal carcinoma in situ (DCIS),** sometimes also called **intraductal carcinoma,** and **lobular carcinoma in situ (LCIS).**

A diagnosis of DCIS is relatively good news: it means that abnormal cells are found only in the lining of the milk duct of the breast, and that these abnormal cells have not spread outside the duct. They also have not spread within the breast, beyond the breast, to the lymph nodes under the arm, or to other parts of the body. DCIS can be found in more than one part of the breast because it travels through the ducts. DCIS has an extremely high cure rate, but if not removed, some types of DCIS may change over time and become invasive cancers. You can reduce your risk of getting the more serious, invasive breast cancers by getting the proper treatment for DCIS.

A diagnosis of LCIS means that abnormal cells are found in the lining of the milk lobule. Although LCIS is not considered to be actual breast cancer at this noninvasive

Noninvasive cancer
cancer confined to its tissue point of origin and not found in surrounding tissues.

Ductal carcinoma in situ
a noninvasive cancer in which abnormal cells are found only in the lining of the milk duct of the breast.

Intraductal carcinoma
see ductal carcinoma in situ.

The Basics

9

Biopsy

a procedure in which cells are collected for microscopic examination.

Mammogram/ mammography

an X-ray examination of the breast.

stage, it is a warning sign of increased risk of developing invasive cancer. LCIS is sometimes found when a **biopsy** (a procedure in which cells are collected for microscopic examination) is done for another lump or unusual change that is found on a **mammogram** (an X-ray examination of the breast; both biopsies and mammograms are described in detail in the following sections).

Because both of these forms of cancer have not spread, their cure rate is high—greater than 90%. They can, however, develop into or raise your risk for a more serious, invasive cancer. If you are diagnosed with an in situ carcinoma, your chances of surviving—and of avoiding recurrence—are very high if you don't wait to treat it. If you do wait, you run the risk that your cancer will become invasive, and thus more difficult to treat.

Invasive cancer

cancer that breaks through normal breast tissue barriers and invades surrounding areas.

Invasive (or **infiltrating**) **cancers** are cancers that have started to break through normal breast tissue barriers and invade surrounding areas. Much more serious than noninvasive cancers, invasive cancers can spread cancer to other parts of the body through the bloodstream and lymphatic system, often invading nearby lymph nodes first. Treatment for such cancers (as discussed in the following section on treatment) is generally a more difficult, long-term proposition, but invasive cancers can often be cured nonetheless.

There are several different types of invasive cancers. As with the noninvasive carcinomas, the most common forms of breast cancer affect the ducts and the lobules. The genetic makeup of the cancer cells is generally one key factor in determining how the cancer is treated;

specific therapies are available to treat estrogen receptor positive (ER+) and HER2 positive (HER2+) varieties (described in more detail in Question 30). These cancers are most commonly discovered as a lump in the breast that shows up on a mammogram or is felt by a woman or her doctor during a breast exam (see Question 12). There are also some rare cancers, such as inflammatory breast cancer and Paget's disease, that differ from the more common ductal and lobular carcinomas in that they do not form a distinct mass or lump in the breast.

Inflammatory breast cancer (IBC) is a rare but aggressive type of breast cancer. Its symptoms resemble an infection or allergic reaction, and are often the same symptoms found in some benign breast diseases, which makes diagnosis difficult. The symptoms include the following: the breast may look red, pinkish, or even orange; it may also feel warm. Ridges, welts, pitting, or hives may be present on the breast, and the skin may look like the peel of an orange. Sudden swelling (as much as a cup size in a couple of days), persistent dark spots that look like bruises, and a change in the color or appearance of the **areola** (the dark area around the nipple) may occur. There may also be pain in the breast, which can be either sharp stabbing pains or persistent aches. These symptoms result from blockage of the lymph vessels in the skin by cancerous cells. There may also be discharge from the nipple, and lymph nodes under the arm or near the collarbone are sometimes swollen. Inflammatory breast cancer grows and metastasizes rapidly and is very serious; if symptoms similar to those listed above do not disappear when treated with a round of antibiotics, a biopsy may

Inflammatory breast cancer
a rare, but aggressive, type of breast cancer characterized by symptoms resembling a skin infection or rash.

Areola
the dark area around the nipple.

be necessary to determine whether the problem is caused by a benign disease or by cancer.

Paget's disease

a rare cancer that begins in the milk ducts of the nipple.

Paget's disease, a rare cancer that begins in the milk ducts of the nipple, differs from IBC in that it grows slowly, but like IBC, the symptoms appear to be an infection or inflammation, and it therefore goes untreated until it becomes more advanced. The symptoms include redness, oozing, crusting, itching, or burning of the nipple. Sometimes, there is a sore that will not heal, and generally only one nipple is affected. As with IBC, any time there is a change in the appearance or condition of the breast, particularly if it persists beyond a few days, it should be checked and monitored by a doctor.

Many women mistakenly think that a change in their breast is not anything to be concerned about if there is no lump.

Many women mistakenly think that a change in their breast is not anything to be concerned about if there is no lump, but the fact is, these rare cancers don't necessarily include tumors or lumps that can be easily detected by touch or by mammogram. For this reason, they often go ignored until they reach an advanced stage and, even then, the problem can be misdiagnosed at first. Any sudden change in the breast that persists for more than a few days should be brought to the attention of a doctor and monitored.

6. There are different types of breast cancers, so are there also different types of benign breast problems?

Many breast problems—such as a prominent breast lump, breast pain, or infection—are usually benign (not cancerous). All the same, if you have any of the breast changes listed in Table 1, be sure to have your breasts checked by a doctor.

Table 1 Breast Problems and Their Association with Cancer

Types of Breast Problems	Found Most Often in . . .	Relationship to Cancer
Cyst: A fluid-filled sac that feels like a soft lump or a tender spot	Women ages 30 to 50 and postmenopausal women taking hormones	Typically is not cancerous; does not increase your chance of getting breast cancer in the future. A rare type of cancer occurs in about 1% of cysts.
Fibroadenoma: A smooth, rubbery, or hard lump that moves easily within the breast tissue	Teenagers and younger women; African-American women; sometimes found in postmenopausal women taking hormones	Typically is not cancerous; if the lump contains certain types of cells, you may have a three times greater chance of developing breast cancer. A rare type of cancer occurs in about 1% of fibroadeno-mas.
Cancer: A hard lump that may or may not be tender	Women who are over age 40 years and younger women with a strong family history	
Cyclical: Breast tenderness that varies over the menstrual cycle	Menstruating women and postmenopausal women taking hormones	Not associated with breast cancer.
Noncyclical: Constant pain in one spot that does not vary over the monthly cycle	Women of all ages and ethnicities	Often from a new or enlarging cyst; about 1% of women with noncyclical pain have cancer.
Non-breast-origin pain: Occurs in the chest wall or ribs under the breast	Women of all ages and ethnicities	Not related to breast cancer, but may be another medical problem that should be checked.

The Basics

13

PART TWO

Risk Factors and Prevention

What risk factors are most important in determining my likelihood of getting cancer?

My breasts are always lumpy. Does this mean I have cancer, or that I'm at a higher risk of getting cancer?

How does estrogen relate to breast cancer?

More ...

7. *What risk factors are most important in determining my likelihood of getting cancer?*

Certain risk factors are more important than others. We'll discuss these factors in order of their probable impact.

Age

The biggest single risk factor for breast cancer is age—the wear and tear of living—and, of course, that risk is always increasing. The average age of women diagnosed with breast cancer is in her early 60s. This does not mean that younger women in their 20s, 30s, and 40s don't get breast cancer, because they do; it simply means that, the older a woman gets, the greater her likelihood of getting breast cancer, taking into account other risk factors. All women are different, and not all women over 60 will get breast cancer; they are simply, on average, more likely to get it than women in their 40s or 50s. The statistic mentioned earlier—that 1 in 8 women will have breast cancer in their lifetime—is frightening, but it is a cumulative statistics, covering a lifetime of over 70 years. More specific statistic that account for a woman's age tell a different (and somewhat more reassuring) story: a woman in her late 30s, for instance, has about a 1 in 257 chance of getting breast cancer, whereas a woman in her mid-50s has about a 1 in 36 chance. The risk increases exponentially after age 30, but even in women 80 years old, the chance of developing cancer is roughly 1 in 24. So what does this mean? It means that, as women age, they need to be vigilant about watching for signs of changes in their breasts, because their risk has increased.

The biggest single risk factor for breast cancer is age—the wear and tear of living—and, of course, that risk is always increasing.

Personal History

Other risk factors include details related to a woman's personal history. Chief among these is a woman's past medical history of breast cancer, **ovarian cancer**, **uterine cancer**, or **colon cancer**. It is important to note that this risk is not a risk of developing a recurrence or metastasis of any of these cancers; it is a risk of developing an unrelated, new cancer in the unaffected breast. Women who have had any of these cancers previously stand a much greater chance of having a new cancer develop in their breast tissue.

Breast cancer is also mildly related to the timing of normal physiological processes, such as **menarche** (start of menstruation) and **menopause** (end of menstrual periods). If a woman's menarche occurs prior to the age of 12, or if her menopause comes after the age of 55, or both, she stands a slightly greater chance of developing breast cancer. Similarly, women who have had no pregnancies, or whose first pregnancy occurred after age 30, are at slightly greater risk than women who had a child before this age; moreover, the decision to breastfeed one's children, as opposed to bottle feeding, seems to affect breast cancer risk, with breastfeeding contributing to decreased cancer rates (the longer a woman breast-feeds, the lower her risk of breast cancer). Radiation exposure at any point in her lifetime, but especially exposure related to treatment of childhood cancer occurring in the chest area, can contribute to a woman's risk of developing breast cancer. Postmenopausal estrogen therapy is associated with an increased risk, particularly in those taking a combination of **estrogen** and **progestin**, but the majority of recent studies do not confirm such risk from oral contraceptives (see Question 9). A diagnosis of **atypical**

Ovarian cancer

cancer beginning in the ovaries; sometimes genetically related to breast cancer.

Uterine cancer

cancer beginning in the uterus.

Colon cancer

cancer beginning in the colon.

Menarche

start of menstruation.

Menopause

end of menstrual periods.

Estrogen

female hormone related to childbearing.

Progestin

a synthetic form of progesterone often used in birth control pills and hormone replacement therapy.

hyperplasia, a noncancerous breast disease character-ized by a growth of abnormal cells within the breast ducts or lobules, points to an increased risk of later de-veloping invasive breast cancer.

Family History

Many people believe that breast cancer is a disease that runs in families. Statistically speaking, this is not true; over 80% of women who are diagnosed with cancer don't have strong familial histories of cancer. Neverthe-less, women with a blood relative who has had breast cancer do have a greater risk, particularly if it's a close relative (mother, sister, daughter). The reason for this increase is that there's a chance that the cancer is caused by a **mutation,** or defective copy of a gene, which might also have been inherited by her close rela-tives. A common belief that such cancer genes are only transmitted from the mother's side of the family is also not true; a genetic risk of developing cancer can be handed down on either the father's or mother's side of the family. That's because half of a person's genes come from their mother, half from their father. But a man with a breast cancer gene abnormality is less likely to develop breast cancer than a woman with a similar gene. So, if you want to learn more about your father's family history, you must look mainly at the women on your father's side, not the men.

A woman with a significant family history of breast and/or ovarian cancer has an increased risk of getting these cancers. You have a significant family history if you have two or more close family members who have had breast and/or ovarian cancer, and if the breast can-cer in the family members has been found before the age of 50. A close family member can be your mother, sister, grandparent (on either your mother's or father's

Atypical hyperplasia

a noncancerous breast disease char-acterized by a growth of abnormal cells within the breast ducts or lobules; can signal an increased risk of developing cancer.

Mutation

defective copy of a gene.

You have a significant family history if you have two or more close family members who have had breast and/or ovarian cancer.

Risk Factors and Prevention

side), mother's sister, or father's sister. Your father, brother, or uncle would also be considered close family members if they had breast cancer, but breast cancer is very rare in men. Your family history of cancer can be assessed by a doctor or other health care professional trained in genetics who will determine if you have a significant family history of breast and/or ovarian cancer. Having this information may help you learn about your cancer risk and help you decide if you should consider genetic testing for the known cancer genes. This subject is discussed further in later questions.

Diet and Physical Fitness

Research suggests that a person's diet may affect the chances of getting some types of cancer. Women who are overweight or obese, particularly older women as noted above, also have a greater risk. And although there are no specific foods shown to increase one's risk of breast cancer, numerous studies have shown that high levels of alcohol intake probably increase the risk of breast cancer. In general, the more alcohol you consume, the higher your risk of developing the disease. Women concerned about their risk of cancer should either not drink, or drink in moderation—no more than one drink per day, defined as 16 ounces of beer, 8 ounces of wine, or a shot of hard liquor.

For overall wellness and possibly to decrease risk for developing breast cancer, it is recommended that women consume a well-balanced diet rich in fruits and vegetables. And what constitutes a well-balanced meal? Traditionally, nutritionists have referred this question to the **food pyramid** highlighted in the U.S. Department of Agriculture's dietary guidelines (see the appendix). The USDA guidelines, which are aimed not at

Food pyramid
a guideline developed by the USDA showing appropriate quantities of different food groups for balanced nutrition.

cancer specifically, but at overall good health, recommend low consumption of fats and sugars (not coincidentally, alcohol contains a high concentration of sugars and therefore falls into this category) combined with high consumption of grains, fruits, and vegetables and moderate consumption of meats, dairy products, and eggs. The guidelines were recently updated to take age and activity levels into account, replacing the traditional "one size fits all" pyramid.

One additional note about diet: there have been a number of claims that eating certain foods or taking certain vitamin or herbal supplements can prevent breast cancer, but none of these have been proven to have more than limited effects, if any—in other words, there's no "magic bullet" out there waiting on your grocery store's shelves. In some cases, these claims are based upon studies in laboratory animals, and there's little reason to think that what works in rats will work as well, or at all, in humans. If you're interested in changing your diet to lower your risk of breast cancer, your best bet is to follow the USDA recommendations as closely as possible.

Maintaining good physical fitness through exercise has been suggested as a potential way to lower cancer risk. Although there is no direct evidence that exercise itself prevents cancer, exercise reduces estrogen levels, fights obesity, lowers insulin levels, and boosts the immune system, all of which can aid in cancer prevention. There is some scientific evidence that women who exercise regularly before menopause gain lifelong benefits against breast cancer, and a recent study in Norway showed that even moderate (four hours per week) exercise contributes to lower risk.

Race

Although it is a myth that breast cancer is a "white women's disease," it is true that, in the United States, whites (especially those of northern European descent) have a higher **incidence** compared to nonwhites. Black and Hispanic women have the next highest incidence, with the lowest rates overall occurring in Korean, American Indian, and Vietnamese women. However, the incidence in nonwhites, specifically blacks, is increasing, particularly in women under age 60; in women under 40, the incidence is higher for black women than white women, and African–American women commonly have the highest overall **mortality** of all groups. High mortality of black breast cancer patients is related to the fact that they often are diagnosed with cancer when they've reached a later stage of the disease, which is more difficult to treat. Though it was previously thought that the problem was one of public health awareness—that black women were not being educated in the need for breast self-exams, mammograms, and other early detection strategies—recent studies have shown that this is not the case, and that the reason for the disparity in disease progression and mortality is indeed biological in nature. Black women usually are diagnosed at a younger age than their white counterparts, and cancers of similar stage and grade in black women are often faster-growing, more aggressive forms and require more aggressive treatment than those in white women. Thus, it is important that black women begin active prevention and detection measures at a younger age than white women, even though they're less likely to get breast cancer, because when they do get it, it can be a more dangerous disease. Organizations that promote breast cancer awareness among black women are listed in the appendix.

Incidence

the number of times a disease occurs within a population of people.

Mortality

the statistical calculation of death rates due to a specific disease or cause within a population.

Other Factors

There are other factors that have been studied but found to be either unrelated to breast cancer or inconclusive—meaning they could be related, but no one can say for sure that they are or aren't. Scientific studies of smoking, abortions, and history of miscarriages—all factors proposed as potentially causing breast cancer—have shown no direct links to this disease (although smoking is a known factor in increasing one's risk of developing other cancers). Research into pollution and other environmental factors is ongoing, but so far it has shown little evidence that these cause breast cancer (but, see Question 9 on estrogen). Breast implants, particularly silicone implants, do not appear to have links to breast cancer, but their presence can make it difficult to get an accurate mammogram and thus it increases the possibility that cancer is not detected or is detected at a later stage. A reduced level of the hormone melatonin, which is related to sleeping patterns, has been linked to breast cancer. All in all, most of these factors are likely to have only a moderate influence on a woman's risk, if any.

8. My breasts are always lumpy. Does this mean I have cancer or that I'm at a higher risk of getting cancer?

Have you ever felt a bumpy texture or "lumpiness" in your breasts? This lumpiness, plus tenderness or pain at certain times of the month, are called **fibrocystic breast changes.** These changes are a normal part of the menstrual cycle. You are most likely to notice them in the premenstrual phase of your cycle or, if you are past menopause, when taking hormones. It's important to do monthly self-exams to familiarize yourself with how your breasts normally look and feel and identify

Fibrocystic breast changes

lumpiness, tenderness, or pain at certain times of the month.

changes if they occur. Fibrocystic changes do not increase your chance of getting breast cancer, and such lumps do not feel the way a cancerous lump would; fibrocystic lumps are softer and more mobile, and there are usually several or many of them that come and go with your cycle. In contrast, a breast lump that should be checked tends to be single, firm, and does not change with your cycle.

Lumpiness is normal for some women. It does not increase a woman's risk of cancer, but it may lull her into a false sense of security: knowing lumps are normal in her breasts, she may be tempted to ignore a lump, particularly if she isn't familiar with normal versus abnormal lumps. For this reason, breast self-exams are important: they're a way of knowing which lumps "belong" and which don't.

9. How does estrogen relate to breast cancer? Can birth control pills or hormone replacement therapy put me at risk?

Cell proliferation

growth and reproduction of cells.

Endometrium

uterine lining.

Estrogen is a female hormone related to childbearing; for this reason, it is most active in the breasts and in the uterus. In turn, the tissues in the breast and uterus are very sensitive to the presence of estrogen. Its job is to prepare the body of an adult woman for pregnancy, which it does by promoting **cell proliferation** in the lobules and ducts of the breast—a precursor to milk production—and in the uterine lining or **endometrium**. During the menstrual cycle, estrogen levels rise following ovulation, but if no fertilized egg gets implanted in the uterus, the amount of estrogen falls sharply, and menstruation takes place.

Because it's a normal element of a woman's physiology, estrogen itself can't be said to cause cancer. However, estrogen's prime function is to speed up the process of cell proliferation; accordingly, estrogen can encourage the growth of cancerous cells once they appear. The more estrogen a woman is exposed to in her lifetime, the greater the chances that estrogen will have the opportunity to promote growth of a tumor. This is why personal history risk factors are so important. A woman who starts menstruating early or goes through menopause late has a longer lifetime exposure to estrogen. A woman who hasn't gone through childbirth or breast-feeding, both of which tend to suppress the menstrual cycle for extended periods of time, doesn't get the risk-lowering benefit of these events.

Today, it is well known that the greater a woman's exposure to estrogen, the greater her risk of developing breast cancer. The effects of **hormone replacement therapy (HRT)** on women who already have breast cancer have not been studied in randomized controlled trials, considered the "gold standard" in medical research. Because more than half of breast cancers are fueled by estrogen, some researchers worry that the use of the hormone could stimulate recurrence of the disease. Improved survival among women with breast cancer has meant that more breast cancer survivors are going through menopause, which for some women causes severe symptoms such as hot flashes, night sweats, and loss of sexual desire. For many years, HRT (usually a combination of the hormones estrogen and progestin) was widely prescribed to women to relieve these menopausal symptoms. It was also thought that HRT might reduce the risk of breast cancer, heart disease, and other conditions. However, in July 2002, a large

Hormone replacement therapy

administration of artificial estrogen and progesterone to alleviate the symptoms of menopause and to prevent health problems experienced by postmenopausal women, particularly osteoporosis.

randomized clinical trial of estrogen and progestin in healthy postmenopausal women was stopped early when researchers found that women who took the hormones had an *increased* risk of developing breast cancer and heart disease. Breast cancer survivors who took hormone replacement therapy (HRT) to relieve menopausal symptoms had more than three times as many breast cancer recurrences as survivors who did not take HRT. It is recommended that women discuss with their doctors whether the benefits of taking estrogen outweigh the risks and that, if used, the hormones should be taken "at the lowest doses for the shortest duration to reach treatment goals."

Xenoestrogens

chemical compounds, usually industrial or pesticidal, that have similar effects in the body as estrogen.

Phytoestrogens

natural, estrogen-like compounds in plant foods, such as whole grains, seeds, fruits, vegetables, and, particularly, soybeans.

There are two other potential sources of exposure to estrogen: **xenoestrogens** and **phytoestrogens**. Xenoestrogens are chemical compounds that have similar effects in the body as estrogen. They are generally related to pesticides and industrial products, such as DDT and PCBs. While both of these compounds are known to be highly toxic to humans and wildlife, no studies have been conducted to determine whether they actually cause breast cancer. It is the opinion of the authors that breast cancer and other cancers of the reproductive tissue would be rare if humans were not exposed to these synthetic hormone-activating agents. Other xenoestrogens have been found to have worrisome effects; one in particular, a compound called diestylstilbestrol or DES, was once given to pregnant women in the 1950s and 1960s to avoid miscarriage. DES, which is no longer in use, was linked to abnormalities of the reproductive organs and an increased risk of breast cancer in children born to mothers who took it.

Phytoestrogens are natural, estrogen-like compounds, or hormone active agents (HAAs), in plant foods, such as whole grains, seeds, fruits, and, particularly, soybeans. Although these HAAs have estrogenic activity, it is between 1/30 to 1/1000 as powerful as natural estrogen. It is thought that it is this low estrogenic activity that makes it protective against breast cancer. Current studies of the effects of phytoestrogens have shown conflicting results; while some indicate the possibility of increased risk, most seem to point toward a substantially decreased risk of breast cancer when women consume foods high in phytoestrogens. Studies to date are inconclusive, but anecdotal evidence regarding the low rates of breast cancer among Asian women, whose diets tend to be high in soy-based phytoestrogens, point to potential benefits. At the moment, it seems likely that phytoestrogens are not a major cause for concern.

10. I've heard a lot of different theories about what causes breast cancer. How do I tell which factors should concern me? Should I do research?

It is important to know the difference between what is a genuine risk factor and what is a myth. Some myths are dispelled simply by knowing what cancer is and how it affects the breast. Knowing that cancer is a process of too-rapid growth in cells tells us that breast cancer isn't contagious; although some cancers are related to viruses (such as liver cancer, which occurs more often in people with hepatitis), breast cancer isn't one of these, so it is not possible to get breast cancer from contact with a person who has it. Nor is it possible to get cancer from a bruise, bump, or similar injury. Hav-

It is important to know the difference between what is a genuine risk factor and what is a myth.

ing large or small breasts neither increases nor decreases your risk of cancer.

When researching cancer, it is wise to be wary of where you get your information; "consider the source" is excellent advice, particularly when searching for information on the Internet. It's not all that unusual for intriguing suggestions about possible "factors" to turn out to consist of nothing more than rumors with little scientific basis. For instance, claims—both published and circulated via e-mail letters—that antiperspirants and underwire bras cause breast cancer by blocking the flow of sweat or lymph fluids are utterly lacking in any scientific evidence to support them, and they're not accurate in their descriptions of the anatomy and physiology involved, either. Such unsubstantiated proposals prey upon the fears and lack of knowledge in the general public and do a disservice to people seeking information.

Even if you're not familiar with medical or academic literature, it's not that hard to determine whether information is valid or not—just use common sense. When someone brings your attention to any information regarding the "cause" of cancer or a "new, dangerous risk," ask yourself, *who is bringing me this information?* If it's your eccentric Aunt Edna (and she's not an oncology specialist), you probably should double-check what she tells you by searching the medical literature. Any reputable paper or Web site should give the authors' credentials; if the credentials aren't there, it may be because the authors are hiding their lack of reliability. Check to see whether the author is affiliated with a university or research institution; look at whether the "warnings" about the "causes" of cancer include vague statements containing words like "might" or "could"; ask yourself whether the authors are implying that something is true rather than offering a hypothesis that they can back up with scientific data, or whether they are stating something as fact, but failing to tell you how they know it's true. Did they perform a **clinical trial**— a study of a drug or treatment with a large group of people testing the treatment? If so, they should state up front where it took place, when it started, how long it lasted, and what number of people were involved. If they don't give this information, consider the results of this "trial" to be suspect information, particularly if you find no mention of it in your other sources. If the trial consisted of a small number of patients—less than 100 is a good rule of thumb—and if there weren't any "control" patients (that is, people taking either placebos or a therapy of known effectiveness) the conclusions in this trial may not be valid or useful.

As a rule, any sources that "sound the alarm!" but do not cite credible, published evidence (preferably in a recognized medical or science forum) should be regarded with extreme skepticism. Always check with reliable sources such as the National Cancer Institute, the American Cancer Society, or the Susan G. Komen Foundation if you're unsure about something you've heard. If there really is a proven, dangerous source of cancer risk, it will be reported by the cancer news services, especially the above-named resources, within days of its announcement. There are also a number of Web sites that specialize in debunking Internet or e-mail hoaxes; a visit to one of those can save you hours of searching on a dead-end topic.

Clinical trial

a study of a drug or treatment with a large group of people testing the treatment.

11. Is there anything I can do to prevent breast cancer?

Most of the associated risk factors cannot be controlled, therefore there are no means of **primary prevention**; that is, there's no vaccine or drug specifically targeted at breast cancer that can make it certain you won't get it. In high-risk women, the drugs tamoxifen and anastrozole are used for preventing recurrent breast cancer. Currently, both are used to treat people with breast cancer. However, **secondary prevention** (limiting the impact of factors you can control, as well as screening for cancer), early detection, and appropriate treatment early in the disease process can help to increase your chances of survival and complete cure should you get cancer. Secondary prevention includes routine breast self-exams beginning around age 20 and screening mammography starting at age 35 to 40, depending on your other risk factors.

Primary prevention

any treatment method or lifestyle change that directly prevents cancer cells from forming, growing, or multiplying.

Secondary prevention

treatments or lifestyle changes that limit a person's exposure to cancer risk factors, but don't directly prevent the formation of cancer.

12. What is a breast self-examination (BSE), and why should I perform one? When should I start doing BSEs? How often should I do BSEs?

A breast self-exam is a way for you to learn the normal look and feel of your breasts and to check for changes every month. Many women have a pattern of lumpiness in their breasts, which is normal. But to know which lumps are normal and which are not, it is important that a woman be as familiar with the internal structure of her breast as possible—and the only way to get this familiarity is through regular, repeated examinations of how the breast structures feel through the skin.

Experts recommend that all women begin performing monthly breast self-exams at the age of 20. The best time to perform a BSE is just as your monthly period ends, when any breast tenderness or swelling has dissipated. For postmenopausal women, it should be performed the same time each month. During a BSE, if you discover a lump or notice any abnormal changes in your breasts, see a trained medical professional for a clinical breast evaluation. Most of the time, the lump will be nothing significant—typically it is a cyst or a similar benign condition—but the knowledge that this cyst exists in this particular spot is important as you "map" your breasts by touch.

13. How do I perform a breast self-examination?

Step 1: Begin by looking at your breasts in the mirror with your shoulders straight and your arms on your hips.

Here's what you should look for:

✔ Breasts that are their usual size, shape, and color
✔ Breasts that are evenly shaped without visible distortion or swelling

If you see any of the following changes, bring them to your doctor's attention:

✔ Dimpling, puckering, or bulging of the skin
✔ A nipple that has changed position or become inverted (pushed inward instead of sticking out)
✔ Redness, soreness, rash, or swelling

Step 2: Now, raise your arms and look for the same changes.

How do I perform a
breast self-examination (BSE)?

Familiarize yourself with the normal condition of your breasts by performing a breast self-examination, as described in Question 13. This exam should be performed monthly, either 2–3 days following your period, or at a specific day of each month if you no longer menstruate.

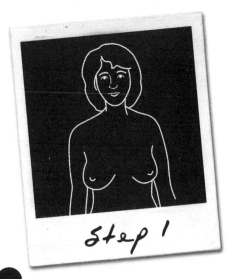

Step 1

1 Stand with your arms at your sides and check your breasts in a mirror.

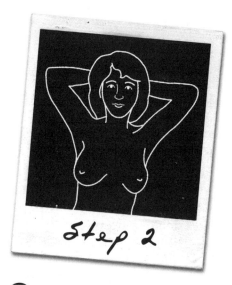

Step 2

2 Raise your arms behind your head and check your breasts again.

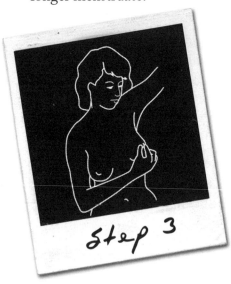

Step 3

3 Gently squeeze nipples to check for discharge.

4 Lie down and, using the tips of your fingers, feel your breasts from top to bottom, including the armpit, using a slow, circular motion. Use both light and firm pressure to feel both surface tissue (light) and deep tissue (firm). If you encounter any lumpiness, make note of where it occurs and what it feels like (whether it's soft, rubbery, or hard, and whether it moves under the fingers or is immobile).

A lump that is new or that has changed significantly in size since your last self exam should be brought to the attention of your doctor.

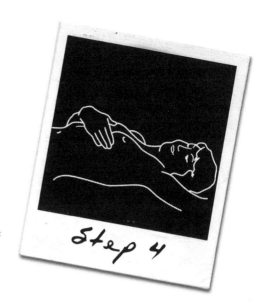

Step 4

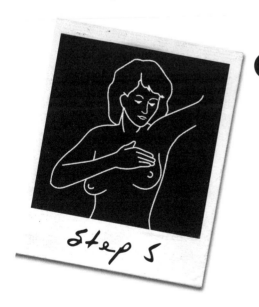

Step 5

5 While standing or sitting, repeat step 4.

Source: **Adapted from the National Cancer Institute**

33

Step 3: While you're at the mirror, gently squeeze each nipple between your finger and thumb and check for nipple discharge(this could be a milky or yellow fluid or blood).

Step 4: Next, feel your breasts while lying down, using your right hand to feel your left breast and then your left hand to feel your right breast. Use a firm, smooth touch with the first few fingers of your hand, keeping the fingers flat and together. This step should be done lying down, not standing or in the shower, because the effects of gravity will work evenly on your breasts in this position. Cover the entire breast from top to bottom, side to side—from your collarbone to the top of your abdomen, and from your armpit to your cleavage.

Follow a pattern to be sure you cover the whole breast. You can begin at the nipple, moving in a larger and larger circle until you reach the outer edge of the breast. Or you can move your fingers up and down vertically, in rows, as if you're mowing a lawn. Be sure to feel all the breast tissue: just beneath your skin (with a soft touch) and down deeper (with a firmer touch). Begin examination of each area with a very soft touch, and then increase pressure so that you can feel the deeper tissue, down to your rib cage.

Step 5: Finally, feel your breasts while you are standing or sitting. Many women find that the easiest way to feel their breasts is when their skin is wet and slippery, so they like to do this step in the shower. Cover your entire breast, using the same hand movements described in step 4.

14. What is a clinical breast exam (CBE)? How often should I get a CBE?

A clinical breast exam is performed by a trained medical professional. It includes a visual examination and palpation (feeling) of the entire breast and underarm area, and is performed in both sitting and lying down positions. Clinical breast exams are recommended for all women at the age of 20, and thereafter every three years, or every year if you are age 35 and over. It is important for women over the age of 40 to have both a clinical breast examination and mammogram each year. Women under age 40 with a family history or other risk factor should talk with a trained medical professional about having a mammogram.

15. What is the Breast Cancer Risk Assessment Tool?

If you're a woman, you're at risk for breast cancer. And with every passing year, that risk rises. But are you at high risk now? The Breast Cancer Risk Assessment Tool can determine that. Developed by scientists at the National Cancer Institute (NCI) and the National Surgical Adjuvant Breast and Bowel Project (NSABP) Biostatistics Center, the Breast Cancer Risk Assessment Tool calculates your chances of developing breast cancer over the next 5 years, and up until the age of 90, based on answers to questions about several known breast cancer risks.

The program, which is available to physicians on a CD-ROM from the National Cancer Institute or can be accessed by anyone from the National Cancer Institute's Web site, uses statistical methods applied to data from a mammography screening project conducted in the 1970s called the Breast Cancer Detection and Demonstration Project. By answering a short series of questions about the patient's most significant likely risk factors—previous diagnosis of DCIS/LCIS, current age, age at menarche, age at birth of first child, number of close relatives diagnosed with cancer, whether or not the patient had any suspicious symptoms requiring a biopsy, and whether the biopsy showed atypical cells—the tool's user can get a statistic demonstrating the patient's risk of getting cancer at five years, over her lifetime, or at any specified age. The caveat to this tool is that it is intended to assist physicians in assessing a woman's risks so they can help her determine whether prophylactic measures such as tamoxifen are necessary. It will generally underestimate risk in women with strong family histories of breast cancer. Thus, if you decide to use this test independently, any results indicating high risk should be discussed with your physician. Even when the test does not indicate high risk, it should be taken with a grain of salt; as the NCI's Web site points out, other potential risk factors "such as age at menopause, dense breast tissue on a mammogram, use of birth control pills or hormone replacement therapy, high-fat diet, alcohol, physical activity, obesity, or environmental exposures are not included in this risk assessment tool for two reasons: evidence is either not conclusive or researchers cannot accurately determine how much these factors contribute to the calculation of risk for an individual woman." The test is a statistical tool only, lacking the ability to assess the complete range of factors for every individual, so it should be used in conjunction with advice from your doctor on how to respond to and minimize your personal risk of breast cancer.

16. Do mammograms prevent breast cancer? Who should get one, and why?

Mammograms do not prevent breast cancer; they are a tool for finding cancer, but they can't stop it from occurring. What these tests can do is detect cancer too small for a woman to feel with her hands. Although mammograms are sometimes used to check a lump that a doctor thinks might be cancerous, they are most useful in screening for potential signs of cancer. A radiologist reading a mammogram can locate signs of possible cancer, such as areas of tissue distortion, masses, significant differences between the breasts, and abnormal calcium deposits, long before there are any symptoms that a woman or her doctor can detect.

The National Cancer Institute recommends mammograms for women over the age of 40 on a 1- to 2-year basis, depending on the individual's personal and familial risk factors; women over the age of 50 should schedule mammograms on a yearly basis. It has been estimated that if every woman over the age of 50 had her yearly mammogram, breast cancer deaths in this age group would drop by 25% or more. Mammograms are also recommended for women 35 and older who have a strong familial history of breast or ovarian cancer—two or more close relatives diagnosed with either of these cancers on either side of the family, particularly if the diagnoses occurred before age 50. Younger women with no significant family history of breast cancer are not encouraged to get mammograms for two reasons: first, breast cancer is unusual in women under 40 when there is no strong family history, and second, younger women's breast tissue tends to be denser and thus more difficult to examine reliably even with X-rays,

It has been estimated that if every woman over the age of 50 had her yearly mammogram, breast cancer deaths in this age group would drop by 25% or more.

so performing the test usually doesn't produce any results worth the expense and time.

17. If mammograms are so good at detecting nonsymptomatic tumors, why should I continue doing breast self-examinations (BSEs)?

At present, regular mammography is the most effective tool available to detect breast cancer. However, mammography is not always completely accurate. (A woman who feels something is wrong with her breast should not assume a normal mammogram rules out a problem. She should discuss her concerns with her doctor.) Mammography cannot reveal every breast cancer at an early stage, and it sometimes arouses suspicion when no cancer is present. Researchers are looking for ways to make mammography more accurate. They are also exploring other techniques to produce detailed pictures of the tissues in the breast. In addition, researchers are studying **tumor markers**, substances that may be present in abnormal amounts in the blood or urine of a woman who has breast cancer. Some of these markers are used to follow women who have already been diagnosed with breast cancer. At this time, however, no blood or urine test is reliable enough to be used routinely to detect breast cancer.

Tumor markers

substances present in abnormal amounts in the blood or urine of a woman with breast cancer.

18. How do genes affect breast cancer risk? Is there a "breast cancer gene"? Does every woman with an altered breast cancer gene get cancer?

Some genes do not function properly because there is a mistake in them. If a gene has a mistake, it is considered mutated or altered. Such **mutations** are not at all unusual; in fact, all people have altered forms of some genes, and most of them are harmless. Some alterations, however, can increase your risk for certain illnesses, such as cancer. Mutations in genes may be inherited or may simply happen to a cell during a person's lifetime. In recent years, gene alterations have been found in some families with a history of breast cancer. Some women in these families also have had ovarian cancer.

There are inherited alterations to specific genes that are linked to about 5–10% of breast cancers. These alterations are most often found in genes named BRCA1 and BRCA2 (BReast CAncer gene 1 and BReast CAncer gene 2). The normal version of these genes does not harm its carrier, but abnormal BRCA1 and BRCA2 genes are associated with higher rates of breast and/or ovarian cancer.

Both men and women have BRCA1 and BRCA2 genes, so alterations in these genes can be passed down from either the mother or the father. Although breast cancer is rare even in men with an altered gene, men with an altered BRCA2 gene have higher rates of breast cancer than men without an altered gene. Men with an altered BRCA1 or BRCA2 gene may also have a slightly increased risk of prostate cancer. Even if a man never develops cancer, he can pass the altered gene to his sons and daughters.

However, having either of these genes does not necessarily mean that breast cancer is inevitable. Although a woman with a BRCA1 or BRCA2 alteration is statistically more likely to develop breast or ovarian cancer than a woman without an alteration, not every woman who has an altered BRCA1 or BRCA2 gene will get breast or ovarian cancer. Genes are not the only factor

Mutation

a gene with a mistake or alteration.

Risk Factors and Prevention

39

*Genes are not
the only factor
that affects
cancer risk.*

that affects cancer risk so an altered gene is not sufficient to cause cancer. Most cases of breast cancer do
not involve an altered BRCA1 or BRCA2 gene. At
most, 1 in 10 breast cancer cases involves an inherited
altered gene, and not all inherited breast cancer involves BRCA1 or BRCA2.

19. What is genetic testing for cancer risk? What should I consider before getting tested? What can I do if I have an altered gene?

Genetic testing looks for inherited genetic alterations
that may be associated with an increased risk of particular
cancers. Genetic testing may reveal whether the cancer
risk in a family is passed through the members' genes.

A woman getting a genetic test provides a blood sample,
which is then sent to a laboratory specializing in genetic
testing. The lab technicians look for alterations in genes
known to increase the risk of breast cancer, such as
BRCA1 and BRCA2. Finding an altered gene can take
several weeks or months, so test results may not be readily
available. The price of testing also varies; it can be quite
high, and it may not be covered by health insurance.

Getting tested for a genetic defect is not a decision to
be made lightly. In addition to the cost, which as noted
can be considerable, the test carries with it both advantages and disadvantages that must be weighed before
making the determination to test. Before you get the
test, it is a good idea to think through why you are contemplating this step, what you hope to learn from it,
and what you want to do with the information, should

you be found to have cancer-related defects. Genetic counselling through a genetic risk program is recommended to understand and sort through these issues before testing.

In most instances, women contemplate testing because they have a familial history of cancer, and they want to know if they or their children could be at increased risk. But the process of getting tested can raise a great many more questions and issues, both practical and emotional. Here's an example: suppose you get the test, and it turns out you have an abnormal BCRA1 gene. What then? You don't actually have cancer, and knowing that you have the gene doesn't tell you when, or even if, cancer will develop in your breast. What do you do with the information you have?

Now suppose you come from a family where you know there's an abnormal gene in your lineage—two of your sisters had the test and came up positive for BCRA1 abnormalities, and your mother and her sister, though never tested, both had breast cancer in their early 50s. There is a fifty-fifty chance that you have this faulty gene too. Do you test for it and find out? Knowing for certain could ease your mind one way or the other, but the test is expensive, and chances are high that you do have it, so why not just save your money, assume you have the faulty gene, and live accordingly? And, how would you cope with it if you took the test and didn't have the faulty gene? Would you be thankful for your good luck? Would you feel guilty that you didn't have to face the increased possibility of breast cancer as your mother, aunt, and sisters do? Would you tell them, or not? If the situation is reversed—you find out you have this gene, but they haven't been tested and have no signs of cancer—what do you tell them? What do you do if they're reluctant to discuss their risk? What if they don't approve of genetic testing or are suspicious of the results you got?

Emotional and family relationship issues are one difficult consequence of the decision to get tested. Even if you feel comfortable with the idea of getting a test, the people around you may not, and there could be discussion and debate no matter what you decide to do. Be aware that getting this test is not the same as going to your doctor's office to get a cholesterol count: what you find out affects not only you, but your children and your immediate relatives, and once you have the information, there's nothing you can do to make it change or go away. And even if you find that you don't have an altered gene, your risk for cancer doesn't disappear—it simply becomes somewhat lower than it would have been if your test had been positive.

What you find out affects not only you, but your children and your immediate relatives.

In spite of all these potential drawbacks, there are good, solid reasons for going ahead with genetic testing. Genetic testing may help you to make medical and lifestyle choices to offset the genetic risk by changing your diet and exercise habits, limiting your use of alcohol, losing weight, and becoming more alert to changes in your body. If you're very concerned about your genetic risk, having the test could relieve your concerns by telling you that you don't have one of these altered genes. Most of all, if you have the test and it is positive for an altered gene, this can tell you that you need to be extra vigilant about screening: a woman who knows she has the mutation for breast cancer has additional incentive to make and keep her mammography appointments—which, depending on her doctor's opinion of her risk level, could be done more frequently—as well as to perform monthly self-exams thoroughly and with care. Furthermore, clinical studies exploring the use of tamoxifen or other drugs as a preventive therapy might be appropriate for people who carry the BRCA1 or BRCA2 mutation; this might be something for a patient and her doctor to discuss should she find that she has this defect, but there may be additional risks associated with these therapies (see Question 53 for more information). Some women with strong familial histories of cancer get the test to help them decide whether **prophylactic mastectomy** or similar preventive surgical treatments are appropriate.

In light of all these considerations, is it worth getting tested? The answer to that question depends on what you expect to get out of the test. The fact is, genetic testing can be beneficial, but there are limitations to what it can do for you. Testing for breast cancer risk will not give you a simple course of action to follow because, although finding a gene alteration in BRCA1 or BRCA2 indicates an increased risk of getting cancer, it does not indicate if or when cancer will develop. Essentially, knowing you have this alteration tells you that you should be even more vigilant about the signs of cancer, and that you are a candidate for the relatively few prophylactic options that are available—but it can't tell you much more than that. It is up to the individual and her doctor to decide whether this information is worth the costs, both monetary and emotional, of having the test done.

If you are at increased risk for breast or ovarian cancer, you can make choices that may help reduce your risk of

Risk Factors and Prevention

Prophylactic mastectomy

removal of a healthy breast in high-risk women to prevent the possible development of cancer at a later time.

getting cancer or help find cancer early. Of course, you can take these steps with or without getting tested for a BRCA1 or BRCA2 alteration.

Increased surveillance: You may choose to be monitored more closely for any sign of cancer. This may include more frequent mammograms, breast exams by your doctor, breast self-exams, and an ultrasound exam of the ovaries.

Prophylactic surgery: You may choose to have your healthy breasts and/or ovaries removed. This strategy is controversial because although it may reduce the risk of cancer, doctors do not know by how much. The surgery cannot remove all of the breast or ovarian tissue, and some women who have chosen this surgery have later developed breast or ovarian cancer in the tissue that was left behind. Thus, choosing to have this surgery may not help you avoid cancer. The ultimate decision is the patient's, but few doctors would recommend that their patients go through this procedure except in women with a strong family history who carry the BRCA1 or BRCA2 mutation.

Join a research study: Because it is not yet possible to prevent cancer, you may choose to join a research study that is looking at ways to reduce cancer risk. This may entail changing your diet, eliminating alcohol, or trying new drugs to reduce the risk of cancer. What is known now about cancer is due in large part to such research. By taking part in a study, you could help researchers find better ways of preventing and treating cancer.

20. Will getting a genetic test affect my health insurance coverage? Can they refuse to cover me if the test is positive?

This concern is a major reason people hesitate to undergo genetic testing: they fear that their insurance companies will discover that they are at high risk and deny them coverage for cancer treatments. Theoretically, if the test is performed by a reputable laboratory and is not paid for by your insurer, there is no reason your insurer or your employer should have access to its results if you choose not to tell them; it is unethical for these results to be shared with anyone other than the patient and the patient's physician (and the latter is bound to confidentiality by standard medical ethics). Your insurer can also have access to documents in your medical record, so if the results are inadvertently placed in your record, the insurer could find out if they have reason to review your complete history. In practice, there have been no documented instances in which insurers have raised rates or cancelled policies on women who had tests for genetic abnormalities, as determined by a study presented to the American Society of Clinical Oncology. The lack of documentation, however, does not allay most people's fears in this regard; what if it's happening, but no one has yet discovered it?

According to the Health Care Finance Administration (HCFA), the Health Insurance Portability and Accountability Act (HIPAA) of 1996 protects you from insurance discrimination based on you or your family's known past or present health status. This means that legally, insurers are not permitted to change your coverage because you had genetic testing performed—the test results are

It is unethical for genetic test results to be shared with anyone other than the patient and the patient's physician.

Risk Factors and Prevention

considered to be a part of your present health status. But employers can establish limits or restrictions on benefits or coverage under a group health plan, so long as those limits and restrictions apply to all individuals in your situation, not just to you. They can also choose to charge a higher premium or request a larger contribution for similarly situated individuals. In addition, employers may change your plan benefits or services if they give you proper notification. What that means is, if after submitting a claim for the genetic test, you suddenly find your company's insurance benefits changed to exclude benefits associated with care of breast cancer, you might have a reason to file a discrimination complaint against your company or your insurer; but if those benefits are excluded with advance notice, prior to your test, and the exclusion is a company-wide exclusion applicable to all employees, there is probably not much you can do about it.

If you are not in a group health plan, and you meet the HIPAA eligibility requirement, you cannot be denied individual health coverage. However, the choices available to you will depend on the approach your state has taken to make health coverage available to you. If you are not an eligible individual, state law rather than HIPAA will determine whether you can be denied coverage. Depending on your state's laws, insurers and HMOs offering individual health insurance may be able to deny coverage based on your health status. Federal laws other than HIPAA and some state laws may ensure that certain people who have lost group coverage are guaranteed access to health coverage, at least temporarily, regardless of their health status.

The National Cancer Act of 2002 requires all insurers to cover the costs of clinical trial participants, as well as expanding Medicare and Medicaid payments for screening, including genetic testing. At this time, it seems likely to pass, so you may wish to investigate its provisions once it becomes law.

21. Where can I get more information about genetic testing? What questions should I ask?

If you are thinking about genetic testing, be sure to talk with your doctor, a genetic counselor, or other health professionals, and take some time to get answers to your questions; some important questions you might have are listed below. You may want to get more than one opinion. For more information on genetic testing or for a referral to centers that have health care professionals trained in genetics, call the National Cancer Institute's Cancer Information Service at 1-800-4-CAN-CER. The Cancer Information Service can also provide information about clinical trials and research studies.

- What are the chances that a gene alteration is involved in the cancer in my family?
- What are my chances of having an altered gene?
- Besides altered BRCA1 or BRCA2 genes, what are other risk factors for breast and ovarian cancer?
- Are all genetic tests the same? How much does the test cost? How long will it take to get my results?
- What are the possible results of the test?
- What would a positive result mean for me?
- What would a negative result mean for me?
- How might a positive test result affect my health insurance? Life insurance? Employment?
- Do I want to submit my test results to an insurance company? If yes, will they pay for the testing?

- Where will my test results be placed/recorded? How might this affect me? Who will have access to them?
- Will having the test do anything to make me change my current health practices?
- What are my reasons for wanting to be tested?
- What type of cancer screening would be recommended if I don't get tested?

Other questions to think about and discuss with your family:

- What effect will the test results have on me and on my relationships with my family members if I have an altered gene? If I don't have an altered gene?
- Should I share my test results with my partner? Parents? Children? Friends? Others? How will they react to the news, which also affects them?
- Are my children ready to learn new information that may one day affect their own health?

PART THREE

Diagnosis

I've found a lump in my breast. What should I do now?

I don't have insurance, but my doctor wants me to have a mammogram to check out a suspicious lump. How can I get a mammogram if I can't afford one?

How is a mammogram performed?

More ...

22. I've found a lump in my breast. What should I do now?

First of all, *do not panic*. Eight out of ten lumps are *not* cancerous. Breast lumps are actually very common, especially in premenopausal women, and they normally go away by the end of the menstrual cycle. But do not ignore a change in your breast, either. The best advice is to consult your doctor or nurse. An examination by a health care provider can confirm the presence of breast changes noted by the patient. The doctor can tell a lot about a lump by carefully feeling the lump and the tissue around it (**palpation**). Benign lumps often feel different from cancerous ones. The doctor may investigate further using any of the following methods:

Imaging

There are several methods by which doctors can look inside the breast to see what is present there and possibly identify a cancerous **breast mass**. The most common imaging method by far is mammography, which uses X-rays to look into the structures of the breast. A second method, **ultrasonography,** uses sound waves instead of X-rays to determine whether a lump is solid or filled with fluid. It can distinguish a liquid-filled cyst from a solid mass, and it can help to distinguish the difference between normal and abnormal breast lumps. A third method, **computerized thermal imaging,** is a much newer technology that analyzes temperature values in breast tissue to measure minute changes in physiological and metabolic activity. It is typically used in conjunction with mammography. A fourth method is magnetic resonance imaging (MRI), approved for use as a supplemental tool, in addition to mammography.

Diagnosis

Palpation

carefully feeling the lump and the tissue around it.

Breast mass

an abnormal collection of tissue within the breast, which may be benign or malignant. A biopsy may be necessary to distinguish benign from malignant masses.

Ultrasonography

uses sound waves to determine whether a lump is solid or filled with fluid.

Computerized thermal imaging

analyzes temperature values to measure minute changes in physiological and metabolic activity.

51

Breast MRI is an excellent problem solving technology. It is often used to investigate breast concerns first detected with mammography, physical exam, or other imaging exams. MRI is also useful for staging breast cancer, determining the most appropriate treatment, and for patient follow-up after breast cancer treatment. While breast MRI is an effective problem-solving technology, it has limitations as a screening tool for breast cancer. Breast MRI's limited availability, expense, and frequent failure to distinguish between cancerous and non-cancerous abnormalities have slowed its widespread acceptance. However, if research continues to show that MRI can be effective as screening women at high risk of breast cancer (particularly young women who have dense breast tissue that makes it difficult to detect with mammography), it may one day play a larger role in breast cancer detection.

Biopsy

When an image of a lump looks suspicious, the next step is usually to try to get some cells from the lump to look at in a laboratory. This is done by one of three methods: **fine needle aspiration biopsy, core needle biopsy,** or **incisional biopsy** of the mass. Fine needle aspiration biopsy (FNAB) uses a very thin needle to collect fluid or cells directly from the mass for evaluation; usually, the doctor performs the procedure while palpating the mass, but if the mass can't be felt easily, ultrasound or computer-guided (**stereotactic**) imaging may be used to assist in locating it. The investigation will either yield fluid, indicating a **cyst,** or it will indicate a solid mass, which may or may not be cancer. If solid, the material removed will be sent to a lab for analysis. FNAB can be done in conjunction with mammography and physical examination with about 98%

Fine needle aspiration biopsy

uses a very thin needle to collect fluid or cells directly from the mass for evaluation.

Core needle biopsy

incorporating a large needle to remove a small cylinder of tissue from the lump for analysis.

Incisional biopsy

removes a portion of the mass for further evaluation.

Stereotactic

computer-guided imaging.

Cyst

a noncancerous, fluid-filled sac that feels like a soft lump or a tender spot.

accuracy in distinguishing benign from cancerous masses. When there is doubt about the results, however, core needle biopsy, incorporating a larger needle, can remove a small cylinder of tissue from the lump for further analysis. In some cases, complete removal of the lump or mass becomes necessary. **Excisional biopsy** involves surgical removal of the entire mass for evaluation, while incisional biopsy removes a portion of the mass for further evaluation.

These tests give one of three results:

- The breast mass is nothing to worry about; return to regular clinical breast exams and yearly mammograms if you are over 40.
- The abnormal tissue probably is not cancer, but return for a recheck in 4 to 6 months.
- A core needle, incisional, or excisional biopsy is needed to tell whether or not the breast change is cancer.

If it is not cancer, your condition may be one of several natural changes the breast undergoes over time. Your doctor will probably recommend that you do monthly breast self-exams and have a clinical breast exam and a mammogram (if you are over 40) every year.

If your breast cells were not cancerous but were not completely normal, you may have a condition that increases your chance of getting cancer. In this case, you would need to have clinical breast exams more often.

If the breast change is cancer, your doctor will talk with you about treatment choices.

Because some of the treatment choices depend on characteristics of the cancer, additional tests may be run

Diagnosis

Excisional biopsy involves surgical removal of the entire mass for evaluation.

on your biopsy specimen to determine whether your cancer has specific traits. For example, a test is usually performed on your biopsy to detect an abnormality called HER2 overexpression that occurs in about 25% of all breast cancers. If your tumor is HER2 positive (i.e., it has HER2 overexpression), your cancer may respond to the drug that targets the HER2 protein (see Question 48 for more on this tumor characteristic and discussion of how such cancers are treated).

23. I don't have insurance, but my doctor wants me to have a mammogram to check out a suspicious lump. How can I get a mammogram if I can't afford one?

A mammogram normally costs anywhere between $50 and $150, and high-quality mammograms can be obtained from a number of providers: breast clinics, radiology departments of hospitals, mobile vans, private radiology practices, and doctors' offices. The costs for yearly screening mammograms are covered under Medicare; if you have not yet had one for this year and you are eligible for Medicare, you can get one at no charge. Coverage for mammograms under Medicaid is available through the screening programs administered through the Centers for Disease Control, which supports early detection programs in all 50 states.

If you are not eligible for either Medicare or Medicaid, there are still a number of options for getting a free or low-cost mammogram:

- The American Cancer Society's national toll-free number is 1-800-ACS-2345, or you can look in the phone book for your local chapter of the ACS. Either the national or local ACS should be able to tell you about any low-cost or free mammography programs in your area that offer mammograms to women unable to pay for it themselves.

- Your state department of health (listed in your phone book) may also be able to help. As many as 20 states now have a **Breast and Cervical Cancer Early Detection Program** funded by the U.S. Centers for Disease Control and Prevention, with more states awaiting approval for funding. This program offers screening to qualifying women unable to pay for it themselves because they have no insurance or are underinsured. If your state does not offer it yet, your state department of health may be able to direct you to other programs that will help you afford a mammogram.

- The YWCA's ENCOREplus Program provides access to low-cost or free mammograms. To find which YWCA facilities offer this service and to learn whether you are eligible, call 1-800-95EPLUS or your local YWCA.

- The National Cancer Institute (1-800-4-CANCER) can provide the names of FDA-certified, accredited mammography facilities in your area. If you explain your financial situation, some mammography facilities are willing to work out a lower fee or payment schedule that will make the test more affordable. Ask the facility's staff if they are willing to discuss these options with you.

- October of each year is National Breast Cancer Awareness Month, and many mammography facilities offer special fees and extended hours during this month. If you happen to need a mammogram at this time of year but need financial help

Diagnosis

Breast and Cervical Cancer Early Detection Program

a program providing low-cost mammography through state health departments.

55

to pay the fees, you might be able to obtain a low-cost mammogram through these programs. However, in a situation where your doctor is concerned about a lump, *don't wait!* If it's not late September or October when this need arises, it is surely not worth jeopardizing your health to lower the costs. Try one of the other methods suggested above.

24. How is a mammogram performed? Is it uncomfortable? Does it hurt?

Mammograms are quick and easy. You undress from the waist up, covering your upper body with a wrap provided by the facility. You stand in front of an X-ray machine, and a technician, generally a woman, will help position your breast on the X-ray plates, flattening it to enable the X-ray machine to get clear a picture of the breast tissue. The pressure of the plates may pinch a little, and the positioning of your body can be uncomfortable, but it usually lasts for only a minute or two, and the whole process of taking the X-ray images lasts about 20 minutes.

You can minimize any discomfort associated with this process by scheduling your mammogram to coincide with the timing of your menstrual cycle. The best time to schedule it would be about a week after your period, and the time to avoid would be the week right before your period, when your breasts are likely to be most sensitive. If standing for an extended time is difficult for you due to other medical problems, make sure the staff performing the mammogram know this in advance—they can arrange to work around your disability. You should also make sure you discuss relevant personal history with the technician, including any prior surgeries, family or personal history of breast cancer, and any new problems or findings in your breasts prior to the X-ray.

There are also certain things you can do to make sure that the mammogram you're going to get is clear, which makes it less likely that you'd have to come back for a second set of X-rays. First, don't wear deodorant or body powder on the day of your mammogram—it can show up as dark spots on the X-rays and interfere with the radiologist's ability to assess the condition of your breasts. Second, be careful to stand perfectly still during the mammogram—if you move, the film could be blurred, and then you'll need to come back. Third, if you've had previous mammograms or biopsies at another facility, bring a list of the dates and locations where these were done; if possible, bring the actual mammograms themselves (it's a good idea to get these from your old facility if you decide to switch to a new one). This allows the physician assessing your mammogram to compare the X-ray to old information, so he or she can better determine if there's anything new or suspicious on the film. Finally, choose your mammography facility with care. At the very least, your facility should have an FDA certificate stating that it meets standards of safety and quality, which should be posted prominently. If it isn't, you have every right to ask to see it, and if they don't have this certificate, you should go somewhere else; any facility without certification is operating illegally and should not be used. If the facility specializes solely in mammography, so much the better—they may be able to perform immediate analysis of your films, so you can have any repeat images made during the same visit if there are any questions about what is seen on the X-rays. If it's possible for you to have your mammograms at the same facility each year, then do it—the longer a facility does your screening, the more familiar they are with your records, and the more likely they are to catch any abnormalities.

If you do not get results immediately, by law you should have them within 30 days of your mammogram; any problems or abnormalities will be reported within 5 working days. Your physician should contact you to give you the results, regardless of whether anything significant was found. If you don't hear anything, don't assume that "no news is good news"; follow up. Chances are pretty good that there's nothing wrong, but don't bet your health—or your life—on what could be a clerical oversight; call your doctor and make sure they give you the results of the test.

Don't assume that "no news is good news"; follow up.

25. What might show up on a mammogram, and what results should concern me?

First, the good news about mammograms: According to the American Cancer Society, only 1 or 2 mammograms out of every 1000 lead to a diagnosis of cancer. Approximately 10% of women will get a report indicating that they need additional mammography, and of these, only 8% to 10% will need a biopsy—and 80% of those biopsies will *not* be cancer.

When a radiologist examines a mammogram, he or she is looking for shadows, masses, distortions, special patterns of tissue density, calcifications, and differences between the two breasts. If none of these findings are reported, the mammogram is considered normal—but if one or more of these findings occur, it's not necessarily an indication of cancer, and, in fact, it's still highly likely that no cancer is present. There are a number of reasons a woman might have an "abnormal" or "suspicious" mammogram, few of which have anything to do with cancer. Mammography is not perfect and there are "false positives" reported—probably about 10% of abnormal results are nothing more than technical or procedural errors. If, for instance, there are technical problems with the film—due to blurs from movement during the X-ray, difficulty in imaging the breast evenly, or even something as simple as a mistake during development of film—the report might come back as "abnormal" with a request for a repeat or follow-up mammogram. The follow-up mammogram should be free of abnormalities if the first report resulted from technical error.

To eliminate the possibility of misunderstanding or oversight, mammogram results have been codified by the American College of Radiology (ACR) so radiologists can measure what they see against a standard to decide whether the abnormality is something to be alarmed about. This system is called the Breast Imaging Reporting and Data System (BIRADS). The numbers help radiologists and physicians to determine whether a follow-up mammogram or a biopsy might be needed. The categories are as follows:

Category 0: Assessment is incomplete and additional imaging evaluation is needed. When the subcategory "/Level 4" is added to the Category 0 classification, it means that a possible abnormality may not be completely seen or defined and will need additional evaluation including the use of spot compression, magnification views, special mammographic views, or ultrasound. A Category 0 classification by itself is nothing more than an inconvenience because the patient must schedule a new appointment, but a Category 0/Level 4 classification is a bit more urgent—it means the radiologist thinks there might be something present, but couldn't see it well enough to be sure. A new mammogram appointment should be scheduled as soon as possible.

Category 1: In this case, there is no significant abnormality to report. The breasts are normal and healthy in appearance.

Category 2: This is also a negative mammogram, but the radiologist viewing the X-ray wants to indicate that there are benign conditions present such as benign calcifications, intramammary lymph nodes, and calcified fibroadenomas. By documenting these conditions, it becomes easier in the future to rule them out as potentially suspicious findings, particularly if the patient should go elsewhere for subsequent mammograms.

Category 3: A Category 3 finding means that there's an area in the breast that is probably benign, but is unusual enough that the physician feels it should be watched. Follow-up with repeat imaging is usually done every 6 months for a year and then every year for 2 years. This approach allows the doctor to keep an eye out for changes that could indicate cancer without subjecting the patient to what is probably an unnecessary biopsy.

Category 4: By categorizing a mammogram as Category 4, the radiologist is recommending a biopsy. In these cases, the results don't definitely indicate cancer, but there is sufficient possibility of malignancy to warrant further investigation.

Category 5: A mammogram listed as Category 5 indicates that there are findings on the X-ray that are characteristic of cancers and have a high probability of malignancy. By putting a mammogram in this category, the radiologist is strongly recommending a biopsy and is sending a message to the primary care physician that immediate investigation and treatment of the lump or mass are necessary.

Characteristics of the mass's appearance can determine whether there's cause for concern. A result of Category 0 or 1 is no cause for concern at all, although a Category 0 result is roughly equivalent to no mammogram and requires a repeat mammogram (unless, as noted above, it's combined with a "/Level 4" finding). Mammography results of Category 2 or 3, in which a biopsy is not recommended by the radiologist, can be caused by any number of conditions, most of which are benign. For example, a common abnormality that shows up as small white specks are **calcifications,** which are tiny mineral deposits in the breast tissue. These come in different sizes and are generally characterized as one of two types, **macrocalcifications** or **microcalcifications.** The pattern of these calcifications is one clue that radiologists use to determine how the mammogram should be categorized. Mammograms also detect noncancerous masses, including **intramammary lymph nodes**, which are normal lymph structures within the breasts, and cysts—small areas or sacs filled with fluid. Cysts, which usually are of little concern but can occasionally become uncomfortable if they become large,

Diagnosis

Calcifications

tiny mineral deposits in the breast tissue.

Macrocalcifications

large calcium deposits in the breast that appear on mammograms as spots within the breast tissue.

Microcalcifications

very small calcium deposits that appear on mammograms as tiny flecks.

Intramammary lymph nodes

normal lymph structures within the breasts.

don't indicate cancer as a rule. Large cysts can be drained if they become painful, but they often grow back; nevertheless, it is very rare that cysts within a breast are connected with malignancy. Alternatively, a mass may be solid, but noncancerous in nature—a thickening of fibrous tissue that feels rubbery and firm, but which isn't a tumor, isn't growing at the rapid pace characteristic of cancerous masses, and isn't in danger of invading other tissues. Such thick areas, referred to as **fibrosis**, require no special treatment—it's enough for a woman and her doctor to be aware they exist so they aren't mistaken for cancerous lumps. All of these findings would fall within Category 2 or 3 and would not require a biopsy.

Fibrosis

thickening of fibrous tissue into a solid mass.

Category 4 or 5 findings are usually triggered by a small number of very specific findings. Clusters of calcifications can indicate the presence of cancer, depending on the shape and density of the clusters. In particular, clusters of microcalcification are often associated with DCIS and are a common sign that cancer is present or may develop. Nearly half of all cancers found by mammography are identified by microcalcification clustering, so findings of such clusters may trigger a Category 4 classification. Also, the presence of masses that are irregular or star shaped will usually alert a radiologist to categorize the mammogram as a 4 or a 5; such irregular shapes are generally indicative of cancer.

26. Why do I need a biopsy if a mammogram has located a mass?

Because symptoms or appearance of benign breast conditions sometimes mimic malignant conditions, it is important to confirm one way or the other which is present. There are also some "in-between" conditions that can only be confirmed by biopsy—conditions that are not cancer, but that can signal the potential risk of cancer and alert a woman and her physician to watch for malignancies. Both typical and atypical forms of **epithelial hyperplasia,** a disease in which the cells lining the ducts or the lobules proliferate, indicate an increase in the risk of cancer; women with typical hyperplasia have a slight (1.5–2 times) increase of developing cancer, while women with atypical hyperplasia have a moderate (4–5 times) increase in risk. Another condition called **adenosis**, which refers to an enlargement of breast lobules, generally creates a lumpy feeling within the breasts, but is not cancerous; there is a slight (1.5–2 times) increase in risk to women with adenosis.

Biopsies from breast masses are examined under a microscope by a **pathologist**, a specialist trained to distinguish normal from abnormal cells. The pathologist's examination determines whether the masses found in a mammogram are simple cysts or something more suspicious; this analysis confirms one way or the other whether the mass contains benign, precancerous, or cancerous cells. The choices for treatment depend on what the pathologist finds in the tissue from the biopsy.

Epithelial hyperplasia

a disease in which the cells lining the ducts or the lobules proliferate.

Adenosis

an enlargement of breast lobules.

Pathologist

a specialist trained to distinguish normal from abnormal cells.

Diagnosis

PART FOUR

Treatment

What should I do if it turns out I *do* have cancer?

What options are available for the treatment
of breast cancer?

A friend suggested I get a second opinion.
Should I?

More ...

Treatment

27. What should I do if it turns out I do *have cancer?*

A diagnosis of cancer is a very difficult thing to accept. Although cancer is no longer necessarily a fatal condition, many people are conditioned to think of it that way. The important thing to remember is, if you do have cancer, you should not wait too long to start treatment. This might seem difficult if you're still in a state of shock from the diagnosis, but there are a number of things you can do to make the process easier and less frightening.

Get a buddy. Many patients find that the information coming from their doctor is overwhelming, and even when they write down what the doctor tells them, they can't clearly recall what they were told they needed to do. If you have a close friend or relative who is willing and able to join you at your consultations—someone with whom you feel very comfortable, as some of the things that will be discussed are very intimate—have that person bring a notepad and pen to take notes for you. If this is not possible, bring a small handheld tape recorder and record the sessions so you can listen to them later when you're feeling less anxious. Try to have friends or relatives with you when you listen to the tape, for moral support. In this way, you can make sure that any anxiety you may feel during the consultations does not interfere with your ability to understand your doctor's instructions and recommendations.

Educate yourself—a little at a time. The fact that you're even reading this book means you've made a start in this direction, but the nature of this text limits the information here to very basic discussions. It may seem a bit morbid to suddenly start studying cancer, but there's a very good, practical rationale for educating yourself: if you know what to expect, it will be much less stressful when you actually experience it, because you'll have an idea of why it's happening and what

If you do have cancer, you should not wait too long to start treatment.

If you know what to expect, it will be much less stressful when you actually experience it.

67

comes next. The amount of information available is vast, so don't feel obligated to become an expert overnight—take it a little bit at a time. What you don't get in this volume, you can find from more comprehensive resources listed in the appendix. There are many resources to further educate yourself on breast cancer treatment available from the National Cancer Institute, the American Cancer Society, the Susan G. Komen Foundation, and similar organizations.

Talk to others in your situation. If you have access to the Internet, you can join some of the breast cancer-oriented chat rooms to discuss your condition with other patients and survivors. If you don't, there are many support groups available for cancer patients; your doctor or local hospital should be able to direct you to one that is convenient, or you can find one through the American Cancer Society, Cancer Care, Inc., and similar organizations (see the appendix). Even if you're not comfortable talking at first, it's worth going to these meetings for the simple reason that spending time with others in your situation might give you valuable tips on how to deal with treatment, side effects, personal issues, and other aspects of the disease that you haven't yet encountered.

28. What options are available for the treatment of breast cancer?

Many treatment options are available for breast cancer. Treatment depends on the size and location of the tumor in the breast, the results of lab tests (including hormone receptor tests and genetic analysis), and the stage (or extent) of the disease. Some treatment options are:

Mastectomy/lumpectomy involves surgical removal of the cancerous tissue and a certain amount of the surrounding tissue as well as nodes from the

Mastectomy/ lumpectomy

surgical removal of the cancerous tissue and a certain amount of the surrounding tissue, sometimes including nodes from the nearby lymph system.

nearby lymph system. The extent of surgery is determined by the type and extent of the cancer, and it may or may not be accompanied by other types of therapy. Surgery can also include a **sentinel node biopsy**, involving removal of the lymph nodes nearest the breast, or an **axillary lymph node dissection**, in which multiple lymph nodes are removed if there is evidence that the cancer has already spread there.

Radiation therapy incorporates the use of high-energy X-rays to kill cancer cells and shrink tumors. Radiation may come from a machine outside the body (external radiation therapy) or from putting materials that produce radiation (radioisotopes) through thin plastic tubes into the area where the cancer cells are found (internal radiation therapy).

Chemotherapy uses drugs to systemically treat cancer. These drugs are provided either orally or intravenously.

Hormonal therapy is used for specific types of cancers that are dependent upon estrogen or progesterone. Hormone therapy works by affecting the way hormones in the body help cancers grow. It can be administered either by using drugs such as anti-estrogens or aromatase inhibitors to block the actions or reduce the amount of these hormones, or by surgical removal of organs that produce hormones, such as the ovaries.

Targeted therapy alters certain types of cell activities within cancerous cells in order to slow or halt tumor growth. One example of this in breast cancer is trastuzumab (Herceptin), which affects a protein called HER2. The HER2 protein contributes to cell growth and development in normal cells; however, some breast tumors have an altered HER2 gene that causes over-production of this protein, promoting rapid growth of cancerous cells.

Treatment

Sentinel node biopsy

addition of dye during breast surgery to help locate the first lymph node attached to the cancerous zone; the node is then removed and biopsied to determine whether cancerous cells are present.

Axillary lymph node dissection

removal of lymph nodes in the armpit during the initial surgery; the nodes are then examined by a pathologist to determine if cancerous cells are present.

Radiation therapy

use of high-energy X-rays to kill cancer cells and shrink tumors.

Chemotherapy

the use of chemical agents (drugs) to systemically treat cancer.

Hormonal therapy

treatment that blocks the effects of hormones upon cancers that depend on hormones to grow (also referred to as endocrine therapy).

Targeted therapy

treatment that targets specific molecules involved in carcinogenesis or tumor growth.

In patients whose tumors have the altered gene, trastuzumab may be used because it is designed to target HER2, and is believed to block its action and impede tumor growth.

The treatments are used under various circumstances; they are discussed further in later questions. There are also a number of other potential options that are still being researched, such as immune system therapies, bone marrow transplants, and peripheral blood stem cell therapies, but these will not be available for patients until they have been proven effective and approved by the FDA. It is worth keeping them in mind, however, because if other treatments don't work well, you might be able to join a clinical trial (see Question 51).

29. A friend suggested I get a second opinion. Should I? If so, how?

Another doctor's opinion often can make your decision about treatment easier. After you receive your doctor's opinion about your diagnosis and/or treatment, you have the right to seek more advice before making any decisions. Getting another opinion is normal medical practice, and telling your doctor you want a second opinion shouldn't offend him or her. Another opinion can help you confirm or adjust your treatment based on the diagnosis and stage of the disease, often helping to ease your mind about your choice of treatment and decisions. Sometimes second-opinion doctors may provide information about a research study that may offer a new breast cancer treatment method or clinical trial.

There are a number of ways you can obtain a second opinion. You can ask your doctor to refer you to another breast cancer specialist. If you're not comfortable with that, call the National Cancer Institute's Cancer Information Service (1-800-4-CANCER) for help in locating cancer specialists that may be in your area; also, talk with women in breast cancer organizations. Ask other women who have been through breast cancer treatment for referrals, keeping in mind that your recommended treatment may be different than theirs, because not all breast cancer cases are the same.

30. What things should I consider when making treatment choices?

A patient's treatment options depend on a number of factors. These factors include age and menopausal status, general health, the location of the tumor, and breast size. Certain features of the tumor cells (such as whether they depend on hormones to grow) are also considered. The most important factor is the stage of the disease. So how do you know what's best for you?

Some options can be eliminated based on the extent and type of cancer you have. If you have early-stage cancer—a small tumor that hasn't spread to the lymph nodes—the full range of treatments is available to you, and perhaps a lumpectomy followed by radiation therapy is the ideal treatment regimen. Multiple tumors, tumors that have gone outside the breast to the lymph nodes, or tumors that have metastasized to other organs in the body must be treated with more aggressive therapies; so while lumpectomy and radiation may still be appropriate treatments, a systemic treatment such as chemotherapy or hormone therapy is also required. Certain types of cancers that are **estrogen-** or **progesterone-receptor positive**—that is, that tend to grow more rapidly with expo-

Estrogen-receptor positive cancer

cancer that grows more rapidly with exposure to the hormone estrogen.

Progesterone-receptor positive cancer

cancer that grows more rapidly with exposure to the hormone progesterone.

71

HER2 overexpression

a genetic feature of some cancers in which an alteration to the HER2 gene causes it to produce excess amounts of the HER2 protein.

sure to the hormones estrogen or progesterone—respond well to therapies that block hormonal effects on these tumors by using hormone therapies (more on this subject in Questions 52–54). Still other cancers have a genetic characteristic called **HER2 overexpression**, which can also aid doctors in choosing potentially effective therapies (see Question 48). By determining whether your cancer falls within these categories, your doctor can include hormonal or biologic therapies in your arsenal. But other aspects of your personal situation may limit the treatment options as determined by the type of cancer you have. For instance, if your overall health is not good—you have heart disease, anemia, or osteoporosis—and you're taking medications for these other conditions, this could also affect whether or not you could tolerate radiation or chemotherapy. Another consideration is your age: older women who have gone through menopause and have no possibility of bearing or breast-feeding children in the future may have a broader range of options, whereas young women who still want families must consider the effects of the different therapies on their ability to have and feed babies. Some hormone or chemotherapy regimens can reduce fertility, usually temporarily, yet surgery may make breastfeeding difficult, if not impossible (see Question 94). Most doctors recommend that women who want to have children following treatment for an aggressive cancer wait at least two years, which is the general time frame for recurrence—but with less aggressive cancers, you might not need to wait so long, depending on your situation. All of these aspects must be discussed between you and your doctor before determining what treatment is best for your situation.

31. The pathologist's report uses categories of "grade" and "stage" in describing my cancer. What do these mean? Which is more important?

When a biopsy has been examined by the pathologist, he or she will issue a report that includes common classifications describing the cancer. Cancers are classified in two ways: by **stage**, which is a numerical determination of how far the cancer has progressed, and by **histologic grade**, which describes how slow or fast the cancer is growing and progressing from stage to stage. Because the grading of cancers is the least complex method of classification, we'll discuss that first.

The histologic grade assigned to a tumor is a way for the pathologist examining the tumor to describe how cancerous cells are arranged in relation to one another and describes some of the features of individual cells. Grading of cancers uses classification levels of 1 to 3. Grade 1 tumors consist of relatively slow-growing cancer cells that look a great deal like normal cells; these are called "well-differentiated" cells. Grade 2 ("moderately differentiated") and Grade 3 ("poorly differentiated") designations describe cancer cells that are scattered in arrangement, abnormal in appearance, and more aggressive in their spread than Grade 1 cancers, with Grade 3 being the fastest growing and most abnormal type.

The stage and grade of a cancer are unrelated to one another, except that the two categories combined describe the status of the cancer in such a way that the doctor can determine how aggressively it must be treated. A Grade 3 cancer caught at a very early stage,

Treatment

Stage

a numerical determination of how far the cancer has progressed.

Histologic grade

describes how slow or fast the cancer is growing and progressing from stage to stage.

though fast growing and aggressive, has a better prognosis than a Grade 1 cancer that isn't discovered until after it metastasizes. All things considered, the stage of a cancer is still more important in determining the treatment strategy than its grade.

The stage of a cancer is based upon a pathologist's examination of the biopsy tissue. Pathologists determine stage based upon the status of three areas of concern: the size and type of the tumor, whether cancer is present in the lymph nodes, and whether metastasis has occurred. The various categories of these areas, taken from the tumor-node-metastasis (TNM) classification system, are taken in combination to assign a stage. Stage is given as one of the following categories:

Stage 0 (early stage) indicates findings of DCIS, LCIS, or tumorless Paget's disease. No actual tumor is reported, and there are no signs of spread to lymph nodes or tissue beyond the breast.

Stage I (early stage) means that cancer cells are not found in the lymph nodes and the tumor is no more than 2 cm (less than one inch) across.

Stage II (early stage) means that cancer has spread to underarm lymph nodes and/or the tumor in the breast is 2 to 5 cm (1 to 2 inches) across. This stage is subdivided into Stages IIA and IIB. Stage IIA consists of any cancers in which there is either no tumor or a tumor at Stage I size, but lymph node involvement has been found. It also includes cancers between 2 and 5 cm that have no lymph node involvement. Stage IIB cancers are 2 cm or larger and show signs of having spread to lymph nodes, but not to the chest wall or skin.

Stage III (advanced stage) is also called locally advanced cancer. The tumor in the breast is usually large (more than 2 inches across), the cancer is extensive in the underarm lymph nodes, or it has spread to other lymph node areas or to other tissues near the breast. Stage III cancers are also divided into two substages. Cancers designated as Stage IIIA include any tumors fitting the description above, while Stage IIIB is reserved for those cancers that have spread to the chest wall or skin, particularly those that have visible external symptoms such as an ulcer on the breast skin, edema, or "orange peel" appearance of the skin. Inflammatory breast cancer is a Stage IIIB type of locally advanced breast cancer.

Stage IV is metastatic cancer. The size of the tumor and extent of spread to lymph nodes are less important in this case than the fact that the cancer has spread from the breast to other organs of the body.

Women with early-stage breast cancer (0–II) may have the option of breast-sparing surgery (followed by radiation therapy as their primary local treatment), or they may have a mastectomy. These approaches are equally effective in treating early-stage breast cancer. The choice of breast-sparing surgery or mastectomy depends mostly on the size and location of the tumor, the size of the woman's breast, certain features of the mammogram, and how the woman feels about preserving her breast (see Question 36 on mastectomy). With either approach, lymph nodes under the arm generally are removed, except in Stage 0 cases. Some women with Stage I and most with Stage II breast cancer have chemotherapy and/or hormonal therapy. This added treatment is called **adjuvant therapy** (see Question 54).

Adjuvant therapy

treatment given after the primary treatment to increase the chances of a cure and to help prevent the cancer from recurring.

75

It is given to treat the whole body to prevent metastases and recurrence.

Patients with Stage III breast cancer usually have both local treatment to remove or destroy the cancer in the breast and systemic treatment to stop the disease from spreading. The local treatment may be surgery and/or radiation therapy to the breast and underarm. The systemic treatment may be chemotherapy, hormonal therapy, or both; it may be given before or after the local treatment.

Women who have Stage IV breast cancer receive chemotherapy and/or hormonal therapy to shrink the tumor or destroy cancer cells throughout the body. They may have surgery or radiation therapy to control the cancer in the breast. Radiation may also be useful to control tumors in other parts of the body. It is important to emphasize that although Stage IV cancer is a very serious illness and has a worse prognosis than cancers caught prior to reaching this stage, it is not necessarily an immediate death sentence: women can and do enjoy a good quality of life for years after a diagnosis of metastatic cancer, and there are a number of new therapies available that have proven effective against metastases (see Question 52).

32. What is the difference between cancer and recurrent cancer? How is recurrence prevented or treated?

When cancer is found for the first time, it is treated with the intention of eliminating cancer cells from the body altogether. **Recurrent cancer** means the disease has come back in spite of the initial treatment. Even when a tumor in the breast seems to have been completely removed or destroyed, the disease sometimes re-

Recurrent cancer

the disease has come back in spite of the initial treatment.

turns because undetected cancer cells remained in the area after treatment or because the disease had already spread before treatment. Cancer that returns only in the area of the breast or lymph nodes under the arm is called a **local recurrence**. If the disease returns in another part of the body, it is called **metastatic breast cancer** (or distance disease).

Most cancer patients are screened regularly following the treatment of the initial cancer so that if cancer should recur, it can be caught and treated as soon as possible. Even if the recurrence is detected quickly, however, it could be at a later stage; the treatment determined for recurrent cancer thus may not be the same treatment given for an earlier episode. Patients and their doctors should discuss treatment options for recurrent cancer just as they did for the primary cancer, because the patient may need an entirely new treatment strategy to combat the recurrence.

local recurrence
cancer that returns only in the area of the breast or lymph node under the arm.

metastic breast cancer
cancer that returns in another part of the body.

Treatment

33. Why do I need a team of doctors to treat me? Who are they? How do I choose my team of doctors?

Cancer is a complex disease, and understanding and treating it requires knowledge of genetics, molecular biology, pharmacology, nutrition, and surgery. No one doctor is able to provide all the care and service you may need, so it's necessary to use a team of specialists to look at your case from different perspectives. Your primary care doctor or gynecologist takes the role of synthesizing all of the specific information your specialists discover about your breast cancer and, with the advice of these experts, will help direct you through the various treatments considered appropriate for your care.

Some of the medical experts who may be part of your team are:

Primary care doctor: This is your general care physician, the person who gives you regular check-ups and is likely the person who helped to diagnose you. If your primary care doctor is trained in gynecology, he or she may also act as the manager and main source of information among your treatment team members and you. If not, you may ask him or her to consult with the team if you feel more comfortable having a familiar person on board. Often the presence of someone you know well in your team can be reassuring.

Primary care doctor
a general care physician who gives checkups.

Gynecologist: A specialist in women's health. If your primary care doctor is not a gynecologist, this specialist may manage the team's information, either jointly with your primary physician or as the main doctor heading the team. If you have your own gynecologist who performs your regular exams, you may prefer to ask him or her to perform this function.

Gynecologist
a specialist in women's health.

Nutritionist: A health professional with specialized training in nutrition who can offer help with choices about the foods you eat. Because of the effects that some treatments can have on appetite and nutritional status, it can be important to assess and supplement your diet during cancer treatment.

Nutritionist
a health professional with specialized training in nutrition who can offer help with choices about the foods you eat.

Radiologist: Generally the same doctor who reads your mammogram, the radiologist is part of the team because additional X-rays, such as bone scans or chest films, could be needed to determine the exact stage of your cancer. The radiologist will not necessarily be involved in your treatment, but his or her input is required in determining what the correct treatment should be.

Radiologist
a physician specializing in treatment of disease using radiation therapy.

Oncologist or **medical oncologist:** A cancer specialist who will gather all the information about your case to help determine your treatment choices, including how long, how much, and what types of chemotherapy agents or hormonal therapy are best for you.

Surgical oncologist: A cancer specialist who performs biopsies and other surgical procedures such as removing a lump (lumpectomy) or a breast (mastectomy).

Radiation oncologist: A cancer specialist who determines the amount of radiotherapy required. Not all patients require radiation, so not all teams will include a radiation oncologist, although one should be involved initially to help determine whether you would benefit from this treatment.

Plastic surgeon: A surgical specialist who will perform any reconstruction procedures that might be required, either during or after your breast surgery. This specialist will consult with the oncologists on your team to determine the best timing of such procedures.

In most cases, your primary care physician and/or gynecologist will recommend qualified doctors for each of the positions on your team. Many people simply accept the doctors their primary physician recommends, and if you're comfortable with those choices, then you need not look further than your doctor's recommendations. However, it is usually a good idea to schedule an appointment with at least some of them, particularly the surgical oncologist. You can accomplish this by requesting that your primary physician set up a consultation session in which the surgeon can provide a second opinion on your condition. Because the surgeon usually will be responsible for the first and most difficult portion of your treatment, it is important that you meet him or her and make sure you feel

Oncologist
a cancer specialist who helps determine treatment choices.

Surgical oncologist
a specialist trained in surgical removal of cancerous tumors.

Radiation oncologist
a cancer specialist who determines the amount of radiotherapy required.

Plastic surgeon
a surgical specialist who will perform any reconstruction procedures that might be required.

Treatment

comfortable with his or her qualifications and abilities. The American Board of Medical Specialties (ABMS) certifies specialists, and verification of the physician's credentials can be obtained by visiting the ABMS Web site or calling their toll-free number (see the appendix).

If your primary care physician has no suggestions, or if you aren't comfortable with some of the doctors recommended, your insurance company usually can provide a list of specialists in their database, and you may wish to choose one of these. Another option is to check the list of specialists available from your local chapter of the American Cancer Society or from the National Cancer Institute. There are also a number of online services that can help you to locate both physicians and hospitals accredited to treat your disease—some even provide ratings as to which physicians and hospitals provide the best care. A list of these services is available in the appendix.

34. What is the difference between local and systemic treatment?

Local treatments, such as surgery and radiation therapy, are used to remove, destroy, or control the cancer cells in a specific area. Systemic treatments, such as chemotherapy and hormonal therapy, are used to destroy or control cancer cells anywhere in the body. Depending on the stage the cancer has reached upon detection, a patient may have just one form of treatment or a combination. Different forms of treatment may be given at the same time or one after another. For example, lumpectomy is almost always followed by radiation therapy because a surgeon can't be absolutely certain that all cancerous cells were removed. Chemotherapy or hormone therapy may also be used if it is felt that there is a risk of breast cancer cells spreading to other areas of the body. For larger tumors, mastectomy generally will be followed by a course of radiation and/or chemotherapy to make sure that any metastatic cells are destroyed before they can get a good hold in another part of the body. But it's not always the surgery that comes first: tumors can also be treated with chemotherapy or hormonal therapy to suppress the ability of cells to proliferate, shrinking the tumor prior to surgery.

35. Should I have a bone scan before my breast surgery? What will it tell?

Breast cancer is one of several forms of cancer that can metastasize to the bones. A **bone scan** is an X-ray that looks for signs of metastasis. These are not new cancers, but extensions of the initial breast cancer. If bone metastasis has occurred, it can cause a condition called **hypercalcemia** (accelerated loss of calcium in the bones), which, at the extreme, may leave **osteolytic lesions** (small holes) in the bones. Hypercalcemia and osteolytic lesions can greatly weaken the bones and put the patient at risk of fractures and breaks—particularly problematic for older women who may have already begun to experience loss of bone density (**osteoporosis**) that sometimes comes with age. Other symptoms related to hypercalcemia include nausea, vomiting, and confusion, and while these problems don't weaken the bones, they do weaken the patient and thus present a problem for someone who is already combating a serious illness.

If your initial tumor is large enough to suggest the possibility of metastasis, your physician is likely to suggest a bone scan to ascertain whether to start you on treatment for hypercalcemia. If you have early-stage cancer, a scan might not be recommended, but some metastasis does

Bone scan

an X-ray that looks for signs of metastasis in the bones.

Hypercalcemia

accelerated loss of calcium in the bones leading to elevated levels of the mineral in the bloodstream with symptoms such as nausea and confusion.

Osteolytic lesions

small holes in the bones.

Osteoporosis

loss of bone density.

occur in early stages; if you have experienced aches or pain in your bones, you should alert your doctor to these symptoms and request that a bone scan be ordered. If metastases are found, you will most likely be treated with an intravenous biphosphonate in addition to your chemotherapy and/or hormone therapy to inhibit further bone damage, alleviate common symptoms, and prevent complications of bone metastasis. More information on treatment of this condition is found in Question 48.

SURGICAL TREATMENT

36. What is a mastectomy, and how does it differ from a lumpectomy? Why would I choose one over the other?

Total (simple) mastectomy

the surgeon removes the whole breast but does not remove lymph nodes.

Modified radical mastectomy

the surgeon removes the breast, some lymph nodes under the arm, and the lining over the chest muscles.

Radical mastectomy (Halsted radical mastectomy)

removal of both of the two chest muscles, as well as the breast and lymph nodes.

Lumpectomy

only the tumor and a small section of normal breast tissue are removed from the breast, leaving the breast virtually intact.

Partial mastectomy

a lumpectomy.

The surgical procedures most commonly referred to by the term mastectomy are **total (simple) mastectomy**, in which the surgeon removes the whole breast but does not remove lymph nodes, and **modified radical mastectomy**, in which the surgeon removes the breast, some lymph nodes under the arm, and the lining over the chest muscles. Rarely, a procedure called a **radical mastectomy** (also called Halsted radical mastectomy), in which both of the two chest muscles are removed as well, is used if the cancer is directly extending into the chest wall. Simple mastectomies are used primarily for noninvasive cancers, while modified radical mastectomies are used when there is a possibility of cancer having spread into the lymph nodes.

In a **lumpectomy**, also called a **partial mastectomy**, only the tumor and a small section of normal breast tissue is removed from the breast, leaving the breast virtually intact. There is also a procedure that falls midway between a mastectomy and a lumpectomy called a

segmental mastectomy. In a segmental mastectomy, the surgeon removes the tumor, some of the normal breast tissue around it, and the lining over the chest muscles below the tumor. Sometimes, a procedure called **axillary lymph node dissection** is done in conjunction with the breast surgery. This procedure involves removal of lymph nodes in the armpit during the initial surgery; the nodes are then examined by a pathologist to determine whether cancerous cells are present. Alternatively, the surgeon can also perform a **sentinel node biopsy**, in which a dye is added to the area of the tumor to help locate the first lymph node draining the cancerous zone. The lymph node that is stained by the dye first is removed during surgery to have the pathologist look for breast cancer cells within them. Both lumpectomies and segmental mastectomies minimize the amount of breast tissue taken by the surgeon, and both should be followed by a course of radiation treatment; these therapies are referred to as "breast-conserving therapies" because the goal is to both remove the cancer and maintain as much of the original breast tissue as possible.

Both forms of treatment have their advantages and disadvantages. The goal of surgery is to physically remove all cancer cells from the breast. When tumors are very large or have extremely irregular shapes, modified radical and total mastectomies are more effective in achieving this goal than lumpectomies. However, there are drawbacks to totally removing the breast: in addition to the strain of major surgery on the patient's physical and emotional well-being, the loss of a breast can bring feelings of depression and insecurity, and can inhibit the patient's sexuality (see Questions 86 and 90). In cases where it's medically appropriate, breast-conserving therapy can alleviate some of these potential problems.

Treatment

Segmental mastectomy

removal of the tumor, some of the normal breast tissue around it, and the lining over the chest muscles below the tumor.

Axillary lymph node dissection

a procedure that involves removal of lymph nodes in the armpit during the initial surgery; the nodes are then examined by a pathologist to determine whether cancerous cells are present.

Sentinal node biopsy

a procedure in which a dye is added to the area of the tumor to help locate the first lymph node draining the cancerous zone.

Breast-conserving therapy has proven highly effective for smaller or more regularly shaped tumors that haven't metastasized and is particularly attractive for women who want to preserve their breast as much as possible. Because only a small amount of breast tissue beyond the tumor is taken, radiation therapy is necessary to make sure that any remaining cancer cells are killed; these treatments can require daily (Monday through Friday) outpatient visits for as many as six weeks, with regular additional check-ups afterward. Breast-conserving therapy is therefore a more extended course of treatment than mastectomy. There are also some complications related to axial node dissection, such as lymphedema, that will be discussed in Question 40.

The treatment that is best for you depends on the grade and stage of your tumor and, to a certain degree, upon your personal preferences and priorities. If you are greatly concerned about how your body will look following surgery, you should discuss this with your doctor so she or he will know that this is a consideration in choosing the type of surgery. Your doctor should be able to give you a detailed description of how your body will look following surgery and assist you in determining how to obtain a satisfactory result. Breast-conserving therapy may not be an option for you, but even if that's the case, there are still ways in which your surgeon could assist in restoring your physical shape through reconstructive surgery, either during or following the mastectomy. Questions 38 and 39 address the topic of breast reconstruction, and there are additional resources in the appendix.

New surgical procedures are still being developed. Tests of a procedure called **radiofrequency ablation** on breast tumors, for example, have had encouraging re-

Radiofrequency ablation

use of high-frequency alternating current to create frictional heat within the tumor to "burn" the tumor cells to death without the need to actually cut open the breast and remove the cells.

sults, and studies are ongoing. This procedure, which uses probes that generate high-frequency alternating current to create frictional heat within the tumor, "burns" the tumor cells to death without the need to actually cut open the breast and remove them. Although it is not yet approved for use in breast cancer, it holds promise that surgery for breast tumors might become a less difficult, less invasive procedure.

37. How do I prepare for surgery? What can I expect after surgery, and how long will it take to recover?

Cancer surgery is performed by either a general surgeon or, when one is available, a surgical oncologist, a specialist trained in surgical removal of cancerous tumors. Prior to the surgery, you should schedule an appointment with your surgeon to talk about the procedure, ask any questions, and address any concerns you may have, particularly regarding possible side effects of the surgery, risks, and postsurgical care. In turn, your surgeon will ask whether you are taking any medications and will go over your medical records with you to make sure you're not on medicines that could affect the surgery. After you have discussed these details with your surgeon, you will sign a consent form that says the doctor can perform the surgery.

The hospital where your surgery is to be performed should contact you a day or so before the scheduled admission date to tell you what they want you to bring with you—clothing, medical records, insurance documents, and the like—and whether you should eat prior to coming to the hospital. If they don't, call the hospital's information line; it is important that you are properly prepared for the surgery.

Treatment

*You have
every right to
ask questions.*

If at any time prior to the surgery you are unclear about what you need to do, what the risks are, or what is going to happen, *ask*. If you have trouble understanding the surgeon's answers or if you find that you're still nervous or frightened, ask whether one of the nursing staff can explain matters to you—a nurse may be able to simplify the process so that you can better understand it. Alternatively, some hospitals have a staff counselor or patient advocate who can help you to make sense of what you're about to undertake. Sometimes a visit to a counselor or chaplain can help you to work through your fears prior to surgery, and entering the process in a positive frame of mind will make the procedure and recovery seem easier. The ultimate point, however, is this: you might find the hospital and the surgeon intimidating or frightening, but they are there to care for your health, both physical and emotional. You are the one with cancer, and the one who's having the operation, so you have every right to ask questions, even if you feel foolish or are afraid to do so—but the hospital staff can't help you if you don't tell them you need assistance.

The time you'll spend in the hospital recovering will vary depending on factors such as your overall health and the type of surgery you need. At most institutions, breast-conserving therapy is done on an outpatient basis, and only mastectomy patients are admitted. Thus, many women are able to return home within a day of the surgery, but others require 2 or 3 days of hospital care. Return to normal activities, such as work and household chores, should wait for about 3–4 weeks to allow your body time to heal. Patients having a lumpectomy—with or without a sentinel node procedure—can sometimes resume normal activities within 1 week.

During surgery, your surgeon may place **drains** in the wound area to collect fluid that accumulates in the area of the surgery. These drains usually consist of plastic tubing and suction bottles; the tube runs from under the incision to a bottle outside your body. These bottles will need to be emptied regularly—your doctor will tell you how often—and the fluid measured, and the place where the tube enters the skin must also be cleaned and covered with fresh dressings. You and your caregivers will be given training in these tasks before the surgery, and you should also be provided with written instructions (if you aren't, ask for them; don't rely on your memory). The drains will be removed when the fluid accumulation decreases—usually about 10 days after surgery—and removal is a quick, relatively painless procedure that does not require anesthesia or a hospital stay. At this point, your surgeon will give you arm and shoulder exercises and additional instructions to help you avoid the complication of **lymphedema** (see Question 40).

The time required for recovery from surgery depends on the extent of the surgery, your overall health, and any complications that might arise.

38. I'm not a candidate for lumpectomy, so the surgeon is recommending total mastectomy. Is it possible to reconstruct my breast?

In past decades, women who had mastectomies either did not undergo reconstructive surgery or had their reconstruction done at some time after the initial mastectomy. Current practices, however, have moved toward a far less radical approach: surgeons generally attempt to ensure complete removal of the disease while sparing as

Drains

consist of plastic tubing and suction bottles; the tube runs from under the incision to a bottle outside your body.

Treatment

Lymphedema

a condition in which lymph fluid collects in tissues following removal of, or damage to, lymph nodes during surgery, causing the limb or affected area of the body to swell.

much original breast tissue as possible. When breast-sparing procedures aren't possible, it has become quite common, indeed standard, to perform the reconstruction immediately following the mastectomy, for the simple reason that the psychological benefits are significant. Waking up to a reconstructed breast is considerably less emotionally painful than dealing with the loss, however short term, of a part of one's body. Immediate reconstruction can also shorten recovery time, and the results tend to be cosmetically superior to delayed reconstruction. However, certain clinical circumstances make delays preferable: if there's a chance radiation therapy might be necessary, the patient and the doctor should confer as to whether to wait, since some kinds of reconstruction involving implants are less successful when the patient subsequently undergoes radiation therapy. Also, the condition of the skin covering the site of the mastectomy is an important consideration; where there is a possibility of necrosis—particularly in women who smoke, are diabetic, or have a collagen vascular disease—the uncertainty inherent in their skin's response to surgery could make it wiser to wait for some healing to take place prior to reconstruction. If reconstruction is something you'd like to consider, you should discuss these considerations with your treatment team before surgery so that they can assess whether immediate reconstruction is a good option for you. If you can't decide one way or the other whether you'd like reconstruction, or what kind of reconstruction you want, you're probably better off waiting; your reconstruction can always be performed at a future date with just as successful an outcome.

There are a number of options for reconstruction, and the type of reconstruction recommended by the surgeon will depend upon specific factors that affect each patient. For instance, the risk of cancer developing in the **contralateral** (opposite) breast is an important consideration because, should the patient need to have both breasts treated, the approach to **bilateral** (both sides) reconstruction might be quite different than **unilateral** (one side) reconstruction. It is also worth considering whether it is feasible to alter the contralateral breast to obtain symmetry, although this could interfere with future monitoring; this decision may make a difference in the technique of breast reconstruction chosen. As just noted, the potential need for radiation therapy following mastectomy also affects the type of reconstruction selected. Patients with back problems should not have certain types of reconstruction procedures (TRAM flap, see Question 39) because the use of abdominal wall muscles may increase stress upon back muscles, exacerbating existing problems. It is important that patients understand exactly how their reconstruction will proceed given their particular circumstances.

Contralateral
opposite.

Bilateral
both sides.

Unilateral
one side.

39. What are the options for breast reconstruction, and how do I know which one to choose? Does insurance cover it, or will I have to pay for breast reconstruction?

In the past decade, advances in breast implants have helped women regain their body image and improve their quality of life. The goal of plastic surgery after breast-removal surgery is to restore the breast to as close to its original appearance as possible. Breast reconstruction usually involves at least one operation, which can sometimes be done at the same time as a mastectomy.

The "new" breast can be composed of an artificial (saline-filled) implant, tissue taken from another part of the woman's body, or both. When tissue is moved, the surgeon must ensure that the relocated tissue has an adequate blood supply. This is done one of two ways: through "rotation flaps" in which the muscle and overlying tissues are rotated into place without cutting the original blood supply to the muscle, or as "free flaps," in which the tissue is detached and the blood vessels are sewn to vessels in the new location to establish a new blood flow. There are three operations that can be done using a woman's own tissue: **latissimus dorsi reconstruction**, **transverse rectus abdominus muscle (TRAM) flap**, and **gluteal flap construction**. Each is explained in more detail below. In contemplating which procedure is right for you, you should ask your plastic surgeon whether you can review photographs of average as well as excellent reconstructions to help you understand the potential outcome of each procedure.

Latissimus dorsi reconstruction. The latissimus dorsi is a large, fan-shaped muscle on the back, below the shoulder. It can be used in a rotational flap reconstruction. Because many women do not have as much tissue (fat and muscle) in this flap to match the amount of tissue removed, an implant is placed under the new muscle so that the reconstruction matches the opposite breast. The patient will have a scar on her back as well as on her chest. This reconstruction has the most reliable blood supply.

Transverse rectus abdominis muscle (TRAM) flap. The transverse rectus abdominis muscle (TRAM) flap is also known as the "tummy tuck." During this procedure, one of two muscles from the abdomen, along with skin and fat, is transferred to

---

Latissimus dorsi reconstruction

the latissimus dorsi muscle (muscle on the back, below the shoulder) is used in creating a new breast following mastectomy.

Transverse rectus abdominis muscle (TRAM) flap

a muscle from the abdomen, along with skin and fat, is transferred to the mastectomy site and shaped like a breast.

Gluteal flap construction

a breast reconstruction technique in which part of the skin, fat, and gluteal muscle from the buttocks is removed and grafted onto the mastectomy site.

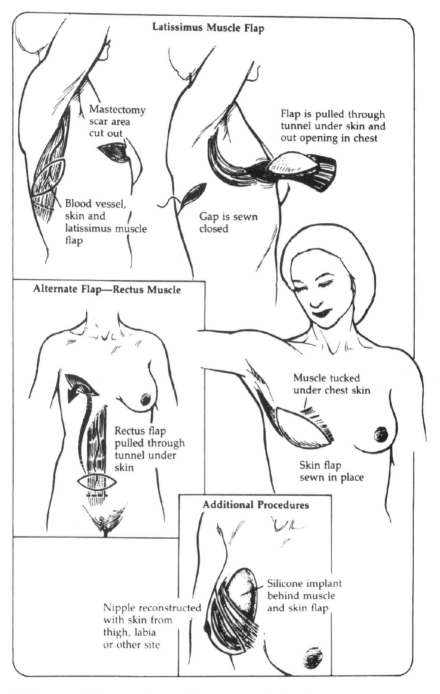

Latissimus Muscle Flap

Mastectomy scar area cut out

Blood vessel, skin and latissimus muscle flap

Flap is pulled through tunnel under skin and out opening in chest

Gap is sewn closed

Alternate Flap—Rectus Muscle

Rectus flap pulled through tunnel under skin

Muscle tucked under chest skin

Skin flap sewn in place

Additional Procedures

Nipple reconstructed with skin from thigh, labia or other site

Silicone implant behind muscle and skin flap

Latissimus muscle flap and rectus muscle flap reconstructive techniques

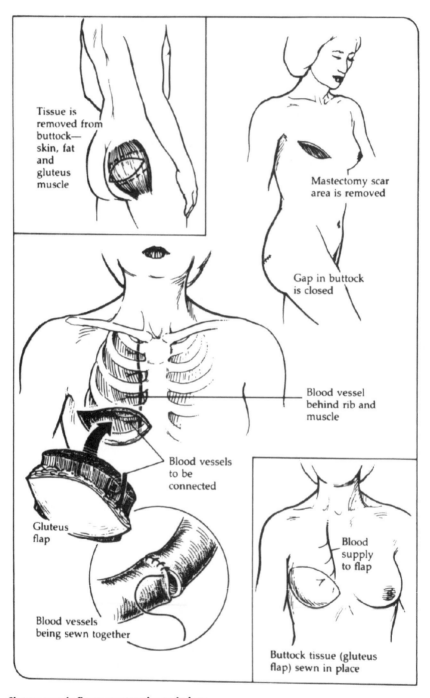

Tissue is removed from buttock—skin, fat and gluteus muscle

Mastectomy scar area is removed

Gap in buttock is closed

Blood vessel behind rib and muscle

Blood vessels to be connected

Gluteus flap

Blood supply to flap

Blood vessels being sewn together

Buttock tissue (gluteus flap) sewn in place

Gluteus muscle flap reconstructive technique

the mastectomy site. It can be done as either a rotational or a free flap reconstruction. This muscle, skin, and fat are then shaped like a breast. Transferring this tissue also causes a tightening of the stomach. TRAM offers a better cosmetic result than the latissumus dorsi, but is more complicated and the blood supply to the reconstructed breast is not as reliable. The patient will have a horizontal scar across the lower abdomen plus a scar on her chest, and the abdominal wall may be weakened.

Gluteal flap construction. The gluteal free flap is a newer technique in reconstructive surgery. For this procedure, the surgeon removes part of the skin and fat from the buttocks and grafts it onto the mastectomy site. The free flap has a higher risk of failure of the blood supply because the vessel feeding the flap is small. Its success depends on tissues getting proper nourishment from the blood vessels.

There is a fourth technique that is newer than the three listed above. This method, called the DIEP flap (DIEP stands for deep inferior epigastric perforator, which is the name of the blood vessels involved), uses fat and skin from the lower abdomen—the same location removed in the TRAM flap—but instead of taking the muscle to bring the vessels supplying the flap, the vessels are dissected from the muscle along with branches going into the fat and tissue being moved. The muscle remains in place, but the tissue and vessels are sewn to the new site.

Artificial implants are also an option if you're concerned about the removal of tissue from other parts of your body. Despite concerns that such implants might not be safe, there have been few documented instances

Treatment

of problems related to saline-filled implants. Implants have the advantage of not requiring removal of additional tissue from your body.

Although it might seem odd to care for a reconstructed breast the way you would your original breast, any original breast tissue left behind is still subject to the same risk factors that were present before your original diagnosis, and you will need to continue cancer screening. A consideration in deciding to use an implant is the fact that the treatment sometimes used to lower the risk of recurrence—radiation therapy—can make reconstruction with artificial implants unsuccessful. If you are considering use of an artificial implant, you should talk to your doctor about these issues.

If your insurance covers mastectomies, then by law it must also cover breast reconstruction. According to The Women's Health and Cancer Rights Act of 1998 (WHCRA), both persons covered under group plans and persons with individual health insurance coverage are covered for reconstruction if they're covered for mastectomies. WHCRA does *not* require health plans or issuers to pay for mastectomies, but most health plans do.

If WHCRA applies to you and if you are receiving benefits in connection with a mastectomy and you elect breast reconstruction, coverage must be provided for:

- Reconstruction of the breast on which the mastectomy has been performed
- Surgery and reconstruction of the other breast to produce a symmetrical appearance
- Prostheses (used by women who are not undergoing reconstruction)

94

- Treatment for physical complications of the mastectomy, including lymphedema (see Question 40)

Whether WHCRA or a state law that affords you the same coverage as WHCRA applies to your coverage depends upon your situation. Generally, WHCRA applies if you are in an HMO. Your state law will determine whether WHCRA will apply to coverage under an insured group plan or to individual health insurance coverage. Contact your state's insurance department to find out whether WHCRA will apply to your coverage if you are not in a self-insured health plan. Note that if you are over 65, have had a mastectomy, and want reconstructive surgery, you may want to contact your local Medicare office. Medicare covers either reconstruction or prosthesis after a mastectomy. The coverage is the same in all states.

40. What is lymphedema, and how is it treated?

Lymphedema (properly called **secondary lymphedema** to distinguish it from the rare form some people are born with) is a condition in which lymph fluid collects in tissues following removal of, or damage to, lymph vessels during surgery, causing the limb or area of the body affected to swell. Left untreated, the swelling can interfere with healing of wounds and perhaps result in an infection, so it's important to watch for signs of lymphedema—and not just immediately following your surgery, as lymphedema occurs weeks, months, or even years later. Lymphedema that appears long after cancer treatment ends can signal a recurrence of the tumor, making vigilance for this symptom doubly important.

Secondary lymphedema

a condition in which lymph fluid collects in tissues following surgical removal of or damage to lymph nodes or vessels.

Lymphedema usually occurs in the hand and arm nearest the affected breast. Fluid accumulates in fatty tissues just below the skin, causing the limb to be swollen and stiff. The symptoms of lymphedema include a full or tight feeling in the limb or skin; decreased flexibility in joints, particularly hands and wrists; difficulty fitting into clothing, especially if this occurs in one specific area; and persistent swelling.

Patients who experience lymphedema are more susceptible to infections.

Acute lymphedema

a temporary condition that lasts less than 6 months in which the skin indents when touched and stays indented, but remains soft to the touch.

There are different types of lymphedema. **Acute lymphedema** is a temporary condition that lasts less than 6 months. The skin indents when touched and stays indented, but remains soft to the touch. The mildest form generally occurs within days after the surgery, and although it is uncomfortable, it's usually not painful. This type of lymphedema is often resolved within a week by elevating the affected limb or by working the muscle or muscles associated with it; for example, performing calf exercises helps alleviate lymphedema in the lower part of the leg. A more severe form of acute lymphedema occurs 4 to 6 weeks following surgery and is considerably more painful because the lymph vessels themselves are swelling. Again, the most common form of treatment is to elevate the affected limb; in addition, your doctor will probably prescribe anti-inflammatory medications to ease the swelling in the lymph vessels. A third form of acute lymphedema occurs slowly and can appear 18 to 24 months or many years after surgery; this is usually not painful, but it is important to be alert to its onset because when lymphedema occurs at this stage or later in the recovery process, it can sometimes indicate regrowth of the tumor or the onset of a chronic problem in the lymph system.

Chronic lymphedema (lymphedema that lasts for longer than 6 months) occurs when the damaged lymphatic system is not able to handle the increased flow of lymph fluid. A number of factors can contribute to the development of this problem:

- Radiation therapy or surgery
- Lack of preventive measures after surgery
- Infection and/or injury of the lymphatic vessels
- Lack of movement of the arm or leg
- Medical conditions such as diabetes, kidney problems, high blood pressure, congestive heart failure, or liver disease
- Tumor recurrence or growth in an area of lymph nodes
- Cancer or cancer treatments that cause loss of appetite, nausea, vomiting, depression, anxiety, or problems with metabolism

Some factors listed here have more scientific evidence behind them than others, but whatever factors might cause it, chronic lymphedema is a serious condition that is very difficult to treat. At present, there are no treatments available in the United States that specifically combat this condition; some doctors in Europe have treated lymphedema successfully with liposuction, but this technique has not yet been approved by the FDA and is still somewhat experimental. Most episodes of lymphedema, whether acute or chronic, are treated through mechanical means (through elevation of the affected part, massage, or use of fitted clothing to keep even pressure on the edema), occasionally complemented with antibiotics to prevent or eliminate infections.

Chronic lymphedema

lymphedema that lasts for longer than 6 months.

Treatment

41. How do I know if I'll get lymphedema? Is there anything I can do to prevent it?

No one can predict who will and who won't get lymphedema, but there are certain circumstances that can trigger it. Infection is one such trigger: patients who have infections around surgical drains or around catheters used for administration of chemotherapy, particularly when such catheters are placed on the same side as the wound, frequently get lymphedema. Even a minor infection can lead to lymphedema, because the lymphatic system is highly stressed after the removal or damage of nearby nodes. In patients using tamoxifen, lymphedema sometimes occurs in the legs. Patients treated with radiation therapy to the underarm area near where the lymph nodes were removed have higher occurrences of lymphedema. Lymphedema is also more common in patients who are overweight or who have poor overall nutrition. If any of these factors apply to you, it's advisable that you keep a close watch for the symptoms of lymphedema and practice some of the preventive measures listed in Table 2, taken from the National Cancer Institute's CancerNet service. (Visit http://cancernet.nci.nih.gov/ and search the Cancer Information–PDQ using the keyword "lymphedema".)

Table 2 Patient Teaching Guide for Preventing Lymphedema

1. Keep the arm or leg raised above the level of the heart, when possible. Avoid making rapid circles with the arm or leg to keep blood from collecting in the outer parts of the limb.

2. Clean the skin of the arm or leg daily and moisten with lotion.

3. Avoid injury and infection of the arm or leg:
   Arms
   • Use an electric razor for shaving.
   • Wear gardening and cooking gloves; use thimbles for sewing.

• Take care of nails; do not cut cuticles.

Table 2 (Continued)

Legs
• Keep the feet covered when going in the ocean.
• Keep the feet clean and dry; wear cotton socks.
• Cut toenails straight across; see a podiatrist.
Either arms or legs
• Use sunscreen.
• Clean cuts with soap and water, then use antibacterial ointment.
• Use gauze wrapping instead of tape.
• Talk to the doctor about any rashes.
• Avoid needle sticks of any type in the affected arm or leg.
• Avoid extreme hot or cold, such as ice packs or heating pads.
• Do not overwork the affected arm or leg.

4. Do not put too much pressure on the arm or leg:
   • Do not cross legs while sitting.
   • Wear loose jewelry.
   • Wear clothes without tight bands.
   • Carry a handbag on the unaffected arm.
   • Do not use blood pressure cuffs on the affected arm.
   • Do not use elastic bandages or stockings with tight bands.
   • Do not sit in one position for more than 30 minutes.

5. Watch for signs of infection, such as redness, pain, heat, swelling, or fever. Call the doctor immediately if any of these signs appear.

6. Do exercises regularly to improve drainage.

7. Keep regular follow-up appointments with the doctor.

8. Check all areas of the arms and legs every day for signs of problems: measure around the arm or leg periodically, or if the limb seems swollen, use a tape measure at two consistent places on the arm or leg. Tell the doctor if the limb suddenly gets larger.

9. The arm or leg may be less sensitive. Use the unaffected limb to test temperatures for bath water or cooking.

10. Eat a well-balanced diet.

Occasionally, patients who travel by airplane experience lymphedema months or years after their surgery;

the cause is probably the rapid increase in ambient pressure that occurs when airplanes descend. To avoid instances of lymphedema, patients are sometimes advised to wear compression garments, such as special sleeves or stockings, when flying to maintain a constant pressure on the arm near their treatment site. It man also help to avoid carrying heavy bags.

RADIATION TREATMENT
42. What is radiation therapy?

Radiation therapy (also called radiotherapy) is the use of high-energy X-rays to damage cancer cells and stop them from growing. Although there are a number of different procedures in development and in use to deliver radiation to the cancer zone (see Question 43), most patients receive **external radiation therapy**, in which the X-rays come from radioactive material outside the body and are directed at the breast by a machine. A less common procedure uses radioactive material placed directly in the breast in thin plastic tubes (implant radiation or brachytheraphy). Because implant radiation is performed less frequently, most of the descriptions in this book refer to external radiation therapy unless otherwise specified. However, this may be changing. A major National Surgical Adjuvant Breast and Bowel Project (NSABP) is comparing brachytherapy over 5 days or targeted partial breast irradiation given over 5 days to the standard 5–6 weeks of whole breast irradiation in women with early breast cancer following lumpectomy. In either case, the radiation is very carefully targeted to affect a limited number of cells—any remaining cancerous cells and a very small portion of the normal cells surrounding them—in order to limit damage to normal tissues. The goal is to kill the diseased tissue while sparing

External radiation therapy

treatment in which X-rays come from radioactive material outside the body and are directed at the breast by a machine.

healthy tissue, so the doctors in charge of your treatment will take numerous steps to make sure only the cancer zone is affected.

Treatment with radiation therapy is supervised by a radiation oncologist, who determines the dose of radiation based on the size and shape of the breast and the location of the cancer. Radiation therapy is also used after surgery to eliminate any cancerous cells that might remain. Post-surgical treatment usually begins about 2 to 3 weeks following surgery. If chemotherapy has been prescribed, radiation therapy may be given prior to the chemotherapy, in conjunction with it, or delayed until the chemotherapy is finished—the decision depends upon the individual's situation, but it's most commonly given after chemo. For external radiation therapy, patients usually go to the hospital or clinic each day, 5 days a week for 5 to 6 weeks; if breast-sparing surgery was used, this treatment will be given to the whole breast. At the end of the treatment time, an extra boost of radiation is often given that focuses solely upon the place where the tumor was removed. The boost may be either external or internal (using an implant). Patients stay in the hospital for a short time for implant radiation. (See Questions 43 and 46 for more information on implant radiation.)

It is important to note here that in the case of external-beam radiation, you will not become radioactive, nor will you pose a threat to those around you; the radioactive energy entering your cells cannot be re-emitted from your body to harm other people's cells. Don't be afraid to hug, kiss, or touch other people, because you can't hurt them. In the case of internal radiation therapy using very high-energy rays, the implant *can* sometimes pose a risk to others—which is why the therapy is given only in a hospital setting, with strict rules about

You will not become radioactive, nor will you pose a threat to those around you.

who can visit you, how close they can approach, and how long they can stay. Once the implant is removed and you're released from the hospital, again, you pose no danger to anyone else.

43. Are there different kinds of radiation therapy?

Within the general categories of external and internal radiation therapy described in Question 42, there are several different methods designed to deliver radiation to the cancer zone. There are even different types of radiation. Depending upon the factors of a particular case, the radiation oncologist in charge can choose from several radiation sources: X-rays, an electron beam, cobalt-60 gamma rays, or, less often, proton or neutron beams. The radiation is applied using a machine called a linear accelerator. The type of machine and radiation chosen will depend on the size, location, and shape of your cancer, as some forms of radiation work better on deep tumors; others, on tumors near the skin's surface.

The timing and frequency of radiation therapy sessions can also vary. The current standard is for a patient to undergo 5–6 weeks of daily sessions with weekend breaks. New studies are testing alternative methods for radiation therapy, as discussed below. In some circumstances a patient may be a candidate for **intraoperative radiation**, in which a dose of radiation is given directly to the tumor site immediately after the surgery to remove the tumor. This therapy may or may not be followed by external radiation therapy once the patient has recovered from surgery. It has the advantage of providing a much larger dose of radiation to the tumor site than external radiation alone. Alternatively, smaller, more frequent doses, called **hyperfractionated radia-**

Intraoperative radiation

a dose of radiation is given directly to the tumor site immediately after the surgery to remove the tumor.

Hyperfractionated radiation therapy

the daily dose of radiation is given in smaller increments separated by 4 to 6 hours.

tion therapy, are sometimes used. In this form of therapy, the daily dose of radiation is given in smaller increments separated by 4 to 6 hours. Though it has its downside—requiring the patient to come to the hospital two or more times each day can be inconvenient and occasionally stressful—the side effects seem to be reduced, and in some tumors the therapy is more effective. Use of hyperfractionated radiation therapy is not commonplace, but it is becoming more widespread for some forms of cancer.

For women with early breast cancer who undergo lumpectomy, there are promising advances in radiation therapy to prevent the cancer from coming back. Studies have shown that partial breast irradiation delivered twice daily for 5 days is as effective as 5–6 weeks of whole breast irradiation. Another technique, Mammo-Site, may do the same thing. To determine this technique's effectiveness, as well as which patients are best suited to receive partial breast irradiation (PBI) by either technique, a large study is being conducted by the NSABP and Radiation Therapy Oncology Group (RTOG). Three thousand women will be randomized to receive MammoSite brachytherapy, interstitial brachytherapy, or 3-D conformal PBI. MammoSite brachytherapy involves the implantation of a small catheter with a balloon filled with salt water, into which radioactive seeds are placed twice a day for 5 days. After the last treatment, the balloon is deflated and the catheter removed. Interstitial brachytherapy is the use of small catheters placed in the lumpectomy area, in which the radioactive seeds are placed twice a day for 5 days, and then the catheters are removed. 3-D conformal PBI is the use of targeted beams of external radiation therapy focused right around the lumpectomy site, given twice a day for 5 days.

Treatment

There are other forms of radiation therapy that may soon be available. A technique called **radiosurgery ablation,** which uses robotic devices and imaging software to target specific areas with high-energy beams of radiation, is in development. One device previously available only for head and neck tumors was recently approved by the FDA for use anywhere in the body. Although this technology is too new to be in even limited use, the ability to target small zones with high-intensity radiation is important because it minimizes the impact of radiation on healthy tissues.

44. How do I prepare for radiation therapy?

Your treatment will be supervised by your radiation oncologist, who in turn has a team of people to help with the treatment sessions: a **radiation physicist**, who makes sure that the equipment is working properly and that the machines deliver the precise dose of radiation; a **dosimetrist**, who works with the oncologist and the radiation physicist to calculate the amount of radiation to be delivered; a **radiation therapist**, who positions you for your treatments and runs the equipment that delivers the radiation; and a **radiation nurse**, who will coordinate your care, help you learn about treatment, and tell you how to manage side effects. The nurse can also answer questions you or your family members may have about your treatment.

Prior to beginning treatment, you will participate in a **simulation** (a practice treatment that allows the team to determine exactly where they want the radioactive beams to be applied). The doctors will review your medical history to determine where to focus the treatment, how much will be required, what type of radia-

Radiosurgery ablation

uses robotic devices and imaging software to target specific areas with high-energy beams of radiation.

Radiation physicist

person who makes sure that the equipment is working properly and that the machines deliver the right dose of radiation.

Dosimetrist

person who works with the oncologist and the radiation physicist to calculate the amount of radiation to be delivered.

tion is required, and how many treatments you should have. They may also take computed tomography (CT) scans to better locate the exact spot to be treated. Once the treatment site (also called a **port** or **field**) is determined, the radiation therapist will mark the target location or locations on your skin, usually with ink. Because the treatment requires you to lie absolutely still, the team may also create molds or immobilization devices to help prevent you from moving—particularly if the position of the cancer means you'll be lying in an awkward or uncomfortable position during treatment. The simulation usually takes anywhere from 30 minutes to 2 hours, so be prepared for a lengthy session; actual treatment sessions are much shorter, about 1 to 5 minutes at most.

45. What happens when I receive radiation therapy? What are the common side effects, and how do I deal with them?

During the actual treatment sessions, you will be asked to change into a hospital gown so that the area to be treated can be exposed easily. The radiation therapist will position you on a table, place shields or blocks over you to protect healthy tissues and organs, and set up any devices created to help you stay completely still. Then the therapist will leave the room, although he or she will be able to see you and talk to you from the nearby room from which the radiation machines are operated. You should expect to see the machines in the room move around—they are being controlled from the next room by the radiation therapist.

The application of radiation takes only about 1 to 5 minutes, and you will feel, hear, see, and smell nothing—the treatment is entirely painless and is similar to

Radiation therapist
person who positions patients for radiation treatments and runs the equipment that delivers the radiation.

Radiation nurse
person who coordinates radiation therapy and patient care, helps patients learn about treatment, and assists in management of side effects.

Simulation
a practice treatment that allows the team to determine exactly where they want the radioactive beams to be applied.

Port or field
the treatment site.

having an X-ray. However, if at any time you feel uncomfortable or ill, you should immediately tell your radiation therapist; the treatment can be halted if necessary. Any other questions or concerns you may have about the session should also be directed to the radiation therapist.

Radiation treatment affects every patient differently, depending on the dosage and on the patient's overall health. That said, it typically causes only minor side effects, and some patients experience none at all. You will be given a list of likely side effects by your doctor or nurse. It's important to make sure that your doctor is aware of any medications you're taking, whether over-the-counter or prescription, or allergies you have so he or she can help you minimize side effects. Also, if you experience unusual symptoms, such as sweating, fever, or pain, tell your doctor immediately.

Most of the side effects related to radiation therapy are not serious, although they can be uncomfortable: skin irritation, redness, itching, and similar symptoms are among the most common. These are temporary, lasting about 6 weeks, and are usually dealt with by practicing the techniques listed in Table 3. You may also have some minor, long-term changes, such as a darkening of the skin in the treated area and an increase in the size of pores in the skin. These changes can last a year or longer after treatment. There is also a condition in which small, red areas called **telangiectasias** appear, caused by dilation in blood vessels of the skin; these, too, should fade in time, although they can be permanent.

Telangiectasias

small, red areas that appear on the skin, caused by dilation in blood vessels of the skin.

Some patients experience loss of appetite and difficulty in digestion during radiation therapy; it is not unusual for patients to lose several pounds during treatment.

Table 3   Techniques for Relieving Skin Discomfort During Radiation Treatment

- Before using soaps, lotions, deodorants, sun blocks, medicines, perfumes, cosmetics, talcum powder, or other substances in the treated area, ask your doctor or nurse if they will irritate the skin. Do not use any of these substances within 2 hours of treatment.
- Wear loose, soft cotton clothing over the treated area. Do not wear starched or stiff clothing over the treated area.
- Do not scratch, rub, or scrub treated skin.
- Do not use adhesive tape on treated skin. If bandaging is necessary, use paper tape and apply it outside of the treatment area. Your nurse can help you place dressings so that you can avoid irritating the treated area.
- Do not apply heat or cold (heating pad, ice pack, etc.) to the treated area. Use only lukewarm water for bathing the area.
- Use an electric shaver if you must shave the treated area, but only after checking with your doctor or nurse. Do not use a preshave lotion or hair-removal products on the treated area.
- Protect the treatment area from the sun.

Adapted from National Cancer Institute/CancerNet: *Radiation Therapy and You: A Guide to Self-Help During Cancer Treatment.*

Fatigue is also fairly common, but it can be alleviated by taking a few simple steps. First, make sure you are getting proper nutrition. If your appetite is poor, you must be especially careful about what you eat, because otherwise you might deplete your energy through poor nutrition. (See Question 49 on side effects.) Fatigue is sometimes related to counts of **red blood cells**, **white blood cells**, and **platelets** in the blood, which frequently drop during radiation therapy and which can also be affected by an unbalanced diet. A second method of combating fatigue is, somewhat surprisingly, engaging in mild exercise—a short walk, for example, can sometimes reduce tiredness. If fatigue is severe or chronic, however, you might want to make arrangements to get assistance in everyday tasks, such as shopping or housework, to reduce the demands on your energy. Some pa-

Red blood cells

cells in the blood with the primary function of carrying oxygen to tissues.

White blood cells

cells in the blood with the primary function of combating infection.

Platelets

components of blood that assist in clotting and wound healing.

tients go to their employers and request limited work hours or take time off during the weeks they expect to receive treatment. Fatigue can last 4 to 6 weeks after treatment ends, so it's important to pace yourself carefully. If you experience stiffness or difficulty moving the arm near your treated breast, ask your doctor for exercises to help alleviate the problem.

46. How does internal radiation therapy differ from external radiation therapy?

Internal radiation therapy differs from external radiation therapy in both the way the radiation is delivered to the body and the overall effects of the therapy. Internal radiation therapy permits a higher dose of radiation to be aimed in a very specific location—the tumor if surgery hasn't yet been performed or the original site of the tumor if it has. Internal radiation can be used either alone or in combination with external radiation therapy or other therapies.

Brachytherapy

a form of internal radiation therapy.

Interstitial radiation

a form of internal radiation therapy.

If your doctor speaks of **brachytherapy** or **interstitial radiation,** he or she is speaking of one of various forms of internal radiation therapy. There are several methods by which internal radiation therapy is delivered. Radioactive isotopes, such as cesium, iridium, iodine, phosphorus, or palladium, are placed within a tube, wire, or catheter and surgically inserted into the body. How this is done depends on the size of the tumor (if the tumor hasn't yet been surgically removed) and its location. Use of temporary implants is the most common method in the treatment of breast cancer, however, and further discussion of internal radiation will assume that this is the method used.

When internal radiation is administered by catheter or by surgical implantation, the procedure requires a local anesthetic—you won't be put to sleep—and a hospital stay for the duration of the therapy. While the radiation is working, you will be kept isolated from other people; visitors will be limited in how close they can approach and how long they can stay, and nurses may use a lead shield to protect themselves while caring for you. You may also notice some tenderness or tightness in the treated breast; these symptoms should go away when the implant is removed. Removal of these implants is done with a local anesthetic and should require only an outpatient visit. Even if you have not also had external radiation therapy, you may notice some of the side effects listed in Question 45. As noted above, if any of these side effects continue beyond about 6 weeks or if you experience any other, more severe problems, you should tell your doctor immediately.

For women with early breast cancer who undergo lumpectomy, shorter more intense treatment is being studied (PBI over 5 days) as described in Question 43. Two techniques that are being used are interstitial catheters and MammoSite catheter balloon. A shorter treatment time means that the cost, both financially and in lost work hours, is much less. More women will complete their prescribed radiation therapy and have less inconvenience.

CHEMOTHERAPY AND HORMONAL THERAPY

47. What is chemotherapy? How is hormonal therapy different?

Technically, **chemotherapy** is the use of any chemical agent to treat any medical condition. If you take cold

Chemotherapy

the use of chemical agents (drugs) to systematically treat cancer.

medicine to soothe a sniffle, you're using chemothera-py. But most people associate chemotherapy with can-cer treatment, and in this context it means the use of drugs to kill cancer cells, whether they are in the site of the original tumor or have moved beyond that site else-where in the body.

Chemotherapy for breast cancer is usually a combination of drugs. The drugs may be given by mouth, by intra-venous drip, or by injection; no matter how it's given, chemotherapy is a systemic therapy, because the drugs enter the bloodstream and travel through the body. It is used for multiple purposes: to shrink a tumor prior to surgery, to decrease the chances of recurrence following surgery, to prevent metastasis by killing any cells that may have moved from the original site of the cancer, or any combination of these three.

Cytoxic

the ability to kill fast-growing cells, both cancerous and non-cancerous, by pre-venting them from dividing.

In general, the drugs used in chemotherapy are **cytotoxic**—that is, they poison frequently dividing cells, both cancerous and noncancerous. These drugs kill cells by preventing them from dividing, which is how cells reproduce themselves. This feature is impor-tant because one of the traits that makes cancer dan-gerous is the speed at which cancerous cells reproduce; stop the reproduction, and you stop the cancer. The flip side of this outcome, however, is that other frequently dividing cells in the body that aren't cancerous—hair and bone marrow cells, for instance—are also damaged by chemotherapy drugs. For this reason, the entire treatment isn't usually given at once, but is given in cy-cles: a treatment period followed by a recovery period, then another treatment, and so on. Because bone mar-row cells are crucial to the production of red and white blood cells, the rest period allows the body the time to repair itself by producing new blood cells. It also gives the patient a break—as explained in Question 49, chemotherapy can be a difficult, unpleasant treatment, and the recovery period helps to keep the patient from getting depressed or emotionally exhausted. The rest period serves another purpose as well: because not all cells divide at the same time, administering chemotherapy in cycles allows normal cells that are damaged to recover before the next cycle (dose) of chemotherapy.

Most patients have chemotherapy in an outpatient part of the hospital, at the doctor's office, or at home. Depending on which drugs are given and the patient's general health, however, she may need to stay in the hospital during her treatment.

What is meant by hormonal therapy? We have discussed the fact that some cancers divide more frequently in the presence of the hormone estrogen. Such cancers are called **estrogen-receptor positive (ER+)** cancers. There are also cancers that respond similarly to progesterone (**progesterone-receptor positive** or **PR+** cancers), and others that respond to either hormone **(ER+/ PR+)**. Still other cancers have no hormonal component at all (ER-/PR-). When your cancer is diagnosed, certain lab tests will be done to determine whether your tumor depends on these hormones to grow. If it does, any cancer cells remaining after your surgery or radiation therapy may continue to grow when these hormones are present in your body. The object of **hormonal therapy** (also referred to as **endocrine therapy**), therefore, is to provide a third line of defense by blocking your body's natural hormones from stimulating the division of any remaining cancer cells. Research has shown that hormonal

Estrogen-receptor positive

cancers that grow faster in the presence of estrogen.

Progesterone-receptor positive

cancers that grow more rapidly with exposure to the hormone progesterone.

Hormonal therapy

therapy that limits or prevents the action of hormones upon tumor receptors.

Endocrine therapy

see hormonal therapy.

therapy can extend the lifespan of a breast cancer patient who has cancer cells that depend on hormones to grow. In adjuvant therapy, it can decrease the chance breast cancer comes back in the same or other breast (contralateral). For those cancers that aren't hormone dependent, it usually has little effect and thus is not used. Table 6 gives a list of commonly used hormonal therapies and their effects.

Here's how it works. The receptors and their related hormones are like interlocking pieces of a puzzle. Only those hormones that are "shaped" exactly right will fit into the receptor; progesterone can't affect a tumor that is only ER+, or vice versa, because its chemical "shape" is wrong for the receptor. In order for the tumor to grow quickly, each receptor must be matched up with the correct puzzle piece—estrogen, in the case of ER+ tumors. Hormone therapy seeks to do one of two things: either it lowers the total amount of estrogen available to fit into the ER+ receptor, so that there are many more empty receptors in the tumor than there is estrogen to fill them, or it mimics the "shape" of the hormone and fills the space in the receptor, blocking the estrogen from matching up with it.

48. What are the drugs most commonly used to treat breast cancer? How do they compare to other treatments?

The drugs used in treating breast cancer fall into several categories: some disrupt the growth of cancer cells and others prevent the cancer cells from reproducing. Still others attach to proteins on cancer cells to cause an immune response—in other words, they "flag" can-

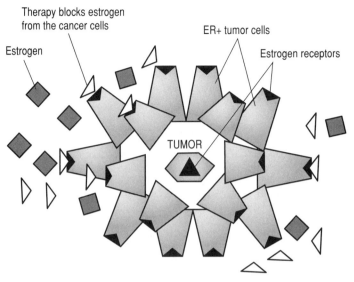

Therapy blocks estrogen
from the cancer cells

Estrogen

ER+ tumor cells

Estrogen receptors

TUMOR

Treatment

cerous cells for the immune system to find and destroy.
Hormone drugs are discussed in Question 52.
Chemotherapy drugs classified as alkylating agents,
anthracycline antibiotics, vinca alkaloids, or an-
timetabolites disrupt cell growth through various
mechanisms. Compounds known as taxanes—so
named because they are derived from the bark of the
Pacific yew tree *Taxus brevifolia*—act upon the reproductive cycle of the cancer cells, preventing division
and causing cell death. Targeted cancer therapy is treatment directed against a specific aspect of a tumor cell.
Therapeutic antibodies engineered through biotech-
nology can be used to target tumor cells. Antibodies are
proteins made by the body's own immune system.
These proteins are directed against foreign or infec-
tious agents. Discoveries in the molecular biology of
cancer led to the development of Herceptin, a biologic
agent that specifically targets the HER2 protein (discussed next and in Table 4).

Table 4 gives a list of drugs approved by the FDA, or being studied, for treating breast cancer. The choice of drugs depends in great part on the type of cancer, its stage, and the patient's overall health. A younger, healthier patient, for example, might be given a more aggressive course of treatment—that is, more toxic, which consequently has more severe side effects—than an elderly or sickly patient whose body might not tolerate the toxicity of the drugs used. Doctors often use a combination of drugs to treat breast cancer, because experience has shown that combination therapies tend to produce a higher long-term survival rate. Particularly when the cancer doesn't have any distinguishing characteristics, such as an affinity to hormones, combining different drugs can "cover all bases" in targeting cancer cells. Using combinations also reduces the possibility that the cancer will become resistant to any one therapy. When the cancer does have such characteristics, they influence the first choice of treatments: for example, about 25% of cancers are characterized by a change in the gene for the **h**uman **e**pidermal growth factor **r**eceptor **2** (HER2) protein, which causes multiple copies of the gene (called **gene amplification**) to produce excessive numbers of HER2 proteins in these cells (called HER2 overexpression). Because the HER2 protein is a growth factor receptor, it can encourage rapid proliferation in cancerous cells with this gene alteration. HER2-positive metastatic breast cancers may be treated with trastuzumab (Herceptin), a drug that targets the HER2 protein.

Gene amplification

a selective increase in the number of copies of a gene, which can lead to the production of higher amounts of a corresponding protein.

A number of drugs are used in varying combinations to treat breast cancer. The most commonly used drugs are cyclophosphamide, methotrexate, 5-fluorouracil, doxorubicin, docetaxel, and paclitaxel. (See Table 4 for details about these drugs.) Other drugs are sometimes substitut-

Table 4   Drugs Used in the Treatment of Breast Cancer

Drug Name Generic (Brand), Maker	Actions / Common Side Effects*
CHEMOTHERAPY	The treatment of cancer using specific chemical agents or drugs that are selectively destructive to malignant cells and tissues.
ALKYLATING AGENTS	Alkylating agents are a group of chemotherapy drugs that target the DNA of cancer cells to prevent the cells from growing or reproducing. Alkylating agents attack cancer cells in all phases and disrupt their growth. These cells are then destroyed.
Cyclophosphamide (Cytoxan) Bristol-Myers Squibb	Cyclophospamide (Cytoxan) is a chemotherapy drug commonly used to treat breast cancer and other cancers. Cyclophospamide first disrupts cancer cells, then destroys them. Cyclophospamide is taken in tablets by mouth or intravenously (through the vein) over 30-60 minutes. **Side effects may include** decrease in blood cell counts with increased risk of infection; nausea, vomiting, diarrhea, and abdominal pain; decreased appetite; hair loss (reversible); bladder damage; fertility impairment; lung and hearing damage (with high doses); sores in mouth or on lips; and stopping of menstrual periods. **Less common side effects:** decreased platelet count (mild) with increased risk of bleeding, blood in urine, darkening of nail beds, acne, fatigue, fetal changes if patient becomes pregnant when taking cyclophosphamide. At high doses, can cause heart problems. Urinary system problems and some secondary cancers have been reported.
ANTHRACYCLINE ANTIBIOTICS	Anthracyclines work by deforming the DNA structure of cancer cells and terminating their biological function. They disrupt the growth of cancer cells, which are then destroyed.
Doxorubicin (Adriamycin) Pfizer	Doxorubicin (Adriamycin) is a type of antibiotic used specifically in the treatment of cancer. It interferes with the multiplication of cancer cells and slows or stops their growth and spread in the body. **Side effects may include** decreased white blood cell count with increased risk of infection, decreased platelet count with increased risk of bleeding, loss of appetite, darkening of nail beds and skin creases of hands, hair loss, damage to the skin if drug gets outside the veins, nausea, and vomiting. **Less common side effects:** sores in mouth or on lips, radiation recall skin changes, fetal abnormalities if taken while pregnant or if patient becomes pregnant while on this drug. Patients should be tested for heart problems before beginning doxorubicin and should be continuously monitored for developing problems during treatment.

*Drug information has been drawn from *The Physicians' Desk Reference*, the FDA web site, CancerSource.com Drug Guide, and, in some cases, specific pharmaceutical companies' web sites. Not all known side effects are listed here; consult with your doctor if you are experiencing side effects, whether they are listed here or not. Many of these medications also have interactions with other medications that produce symptoms not listed here.

Table 4   (Continued)

Drug Name Generic (Brand), Maker	Actions / Common Side Effects*
Epirubicin (Ellence) Pfizer	Epirubicin (Ellence) was approved by the FDA in 1999 to treat early-stage breast cancer after breast surgery (lumpectomy or mastectomy) in patients whose cancer has spread to the lymph nodes. epirubicin helps reduce the likelihood that breast cancer will return and improves a patient's chances of survival. Epirubicin is given intravenously (through the vein) in combination with two other chemotherapy drugs, cyclophosphamide and fluorouracil. **Side effects may include** nausea, vomiting, diarrhea, inflammation of the mouth, hair loss, damage to the skin if drug gets out of the veins, and reduction in white blood cells. **Less common side effects:** There is a risk of irreversible damage to the heart muscle associated with the drug. For women who receive epirubicin as adjuvant therapy, there is a slightly increased risk of treatment-related leukemia. Epirubicin may cause harm to the fetus if taken while pregnant.
ANTIMETABOLITES	**Antimetabolites prevent cells from making DNA and RNA by interfering with the synthesis of nucleic acids, thus disrupting the growth of cancer cells.**
5-Fluorouracil (5-FU, Adrucil, Fluorouracil) multiple makers	5-Fluorouracil is a drug that kills cancer cells by stopping their growth. It can also make it hard for cancer cells to fix damage. **Side effects may include** decreased white blood cell count with increased risk of infection; decreased platelet count with increased risk of bleeding; drowsiness or confusion; darkening of skin and nail beds; dry, flaky skin; nausea; vomiting; sores in mouth or on lips; thinning hair; diarrhea; brittle nails; and increased sensitivity to sun. **Less common side effects**: darkening and stiffening of vein used for giving the drug, decreased appetite, headache, weakness, and muscle aches. Cardiac symptoms are rare, but are most likely in patients with ischemic heart disease.
Capecitabine (Xeloda) Roche	Capecitabine (Xeloda) is approved as a treatment for advanced breast cancer. Capecitabine works by converting to 5-fluorouracil (5-FU) in the body. It is used for cancers resistant to both paclitaxel and anthracyclines. **Side effects may include** diarrhea, nausea, vomiting, loss of appetite or decreased appetite and dehydration sores in mouth or on lips, numbness, tingling, itching of hands and/or feet, skin redness, rash, dryness, decreased white blood cell count with increased risk of infection, decreased platelet count with increased risk of bleeding, decreased red blood cell count with increased risk of fatigue, and irritation of the skin. **Less common side effects**: abdominal pain, constipation, heartburn after eating, fever, sensation of pins and needles in hands and/or feet, headache, dizziness, difficulty falling asleep, eye irritation, and increased value of blood tests for liver function.
Gemcitabine (Gemzar) Lilly Oncology	Gemcitabine (Gemzar) is approved as a treatment for advanced breast cancer in combination with paclitaxel. **Side effects may include** decreased blood counts with increased risk of infection, bleeding, and fatigue; nausea; vomiting; and skin rash. **Less common side effects:** fever, flu-like symptoms, swelling (edema), hair loss, and itching.

*Drug information has been drawn from *The Physicians' Desk Reference*, the FDA web site, CancerSource.com Drug Guide, and, in some cases, specific pharmaceutical companies' web sites. Not all known side effects are listed here; consult with your doctor if you are experiencing side effects, whether they are listed here or not. Many of these medications also have interactions with other medications that produce symptoms not listed here.

Table 4   (Continued)

Drug Name Generic (Brand), Maker	Actions / Common Side Effects*
Methotrexate (MTX, Amethopterin, Folex, Mexate) multiple makers	Methotrexate prevents cells from making DNA and RNA by interfering with the synthesis of nucleic acids, thus stopping the growth of cancer cells. **Side effects may include** nausea (high dose), vomiting (high dose), sores in mouth or on lips, diarrhea, increased risk of sunburn, radiation recall skin changes, and loss of appetite. **Less common side effects:** decreased white blood cell count with increased risk of infection, decreased platelet count with increased risk of bleeding, and kidney damage (high dose). Liver, lung, and nerve damage are sometimes seen with methotrexate use, but the adjuvant drug leucovorin offsets the worst side effects.
TAXANES	**Taxanes are powerful drugs that can stop cancer cells from repairing themselves and making new cells. Often used for treatment of cancers that have not responded to or have recurred after anthracycline therapy.**
Docetaxel (Taxotere) Aventis	Docetaxel (Taxotere) is used to treat advanced breast cancer in patients who have not responded well to chemotherapy with doxorubicin. In 1998, doxorubicin was also approved by the FDA to treat breast cancer that has spread into other areas of the breast or to other parts of the body after treatment with standard chemotherapy. Docetaxel inhibits the division of breast cancer cells by acting on the cell's internal skeleton. **Side effects may include** decreased white blood cell count with increased risk of infection, decreased platelet count with increased risk of bleeding, hair thinning or loss, diarrhea, loss of appetite, nausea, vomiting, rash, and numbness and tingling in hands and/or feet related to peripheral nerve irritation or damage. **Less common side effects:** sores in mouth or on lips, swelling of ankles or hands, increased weight due to fluid retention, fatigue, muscle aches, loss of nails, and redness or irritation of the palms of hands, or soles of feet.
Paclitaxel (Taxol) Bristol-Myers Squibb	Paclitaxel (Taxol) was first approved by the FDA in 1992 to treat advanced (metastatic) breast cancer. In 1999, the FDA also approved paclitaxel to treat early stage breast cancer in patients who have already received chemotherapy with the drug, doxorubicin. Paclitaxel is called a mitotic inhibitor because of its interference with cells during mitosis (cell division). **Side effects may include** decreased white blood cell count with increased risk of infection, fatigue, numbness and tingling in hands and/or feet related to peripheral nerve irritation or damage, muscle and bone aches for 3 days, hair loss, nausea, vomiting, mild diarrhea, and mild stomatitis. **Less common side effects:** allergic reaction: skin rash, flushing, increased heart rate, wheezing, and swelling of face. Transient heart problems such as bradycardia occur in 30% or less of patients and are usually not severe.

*Drug information has been drawn from *The Physicians' Desk Reference*, the FDA web site, CancerSource.com Drug Guide, and, in some cases, specific pharmaceutical companies' web sites. Not all known side effects are listed here; consult with your doctor if you are experiencing side effects, whether they are listed here or not. Many of these medications also have interactions with other medications that produce symptoms not listed here.

Treatment

Table 4   (Continued)

Drug Name Generic (Brand), Maker	Actions / Common Side Effects*
Paclitaxel protein-bound particles for injectable suspension, nanoparticle albumin-bound (nab) paclitaxel (Abraxane) Abraxis Oncology	The nab paclitaxel uses nanotechnology to put paclitaxel in bits of the protein albumin so it can enter the cancer cells more easily. It is used for the treatment of breast cancer that has come back after combination therapy. Higher doses of paclitaxel are given. **Side effects may include** decreased blood counts with increased risk of infection and bleeding, numbness and tingling of the hands and feet related to peripheral nerve irritation, hair loss, muscle and bone aches for 3 days, nausea, and vomiting. **Less common side effects:** fluid retention, and changes in heart test (ECG).
VINCA ALKALOIDS	**A medication in a class of anticancer drugs that inhibits cancer cell growth by stopping cell division (mitosis).**
Vinorelbine (Navelbine) GlaxoSmithKline	Vinorelbine (Navelbine) is used to treat metastatic breast cancer. **Side effects may include** decreased blood counts with increased risk of infection, and damage to the skin if drug gets outside the vein. **Less common side effects:** numbness and tingling of hands and feet, nausea, and vomiting.
TARGETED THERAPY	Targeted therapy is a general term that refers to a medication or drug that targets a specific pathway in the growth and development of a tumor. By attacking or blocking these important targets, the therapy helps to fight the tumor itself.
MONOCLONAL ANTIBODIES (BIOLOGIC AGENTS)	**Monoclonal antibodies work by attaching to a specific protein on cancer cells like a key in a lock, potentially creating an immune response that can help kill the cancer cells. Biologic agents are drugs produced from living organisms or cells. Some targeted therapies are biologics.**
Trastuzumab (Herceptin®) Genentech	Herceptin® (Trastuzumab) is the only FDA-approved therapeutic for HER2 protein overexpressing metastatic breast cancer. Trastuzumab is a therapy for woman with metastatic breast cancer whose tumors have too much HER2 protein. For patients with this disease, trastuzumab is approved for first-line use in combination with paclitaxel, and as a single agent for those who have received one or more chemotherapy regimens. **Possible serious side effects** include development of certain heart problems, including congestive heart failure, severe allergic reactions, infusion reactions, lung problems, blood clots, or a reduction in white blood cells. **Side effects may include:** fatigue, infections, low white or red blood cell counts, trouble breathing, rash/skin blistering, constipation, headache, and muscle pain.
ADJUVANT THERAPY	A variety of drugs that complement the chemotherapy regimen.
Leucovorin	Leucovorin is a form of vitamin used to offset the side effects of methotrexate and/or enhance the action of 5-FU. Leucovorin has few side effects itself, but its use with 5-FU can sometimes exacerbate the side effects of that drug.

*Drug information has been drawn from *The Physicians' Desk Reference*, the FDA web site, CancerSource.com Drug Guide, and, in some cases, specific pharmaceutical companies' web sites. Not all known side effects are listed here; consult with your doctor if you are experiencing side effects, whether they are listed here or not. Many of these medications also have interactions with other medications that produce symptoms not listed here.

Table 4   (Continued)

Drug Name Generic (Brand), Maker	Actions / Common Side Effects*
Pamidronate (Aredia) Novartis Zoledronic acid (Zometa) Novartis	Both drugs are used to alleviate hypercalcemia; zoledronic acid is a newer, more powerful agent. **Both drugs have similar side effects, which may include** fever lasting for a short time (24–48 hours after infusion), pain at place of injection, and irritation of the vein used for giving the drug. **Less common side effects:** nausea, constipation, anemia, and decreased appetite. Renal function should be monitored with use of zoledronic acid. Zoledronic acid can cause bone damage (osteonecrosis) in the jaw.
ANTIEMETICS (ANTINAUSEA)	**Drugs used to prevent nausea or vomiting. Antiemetics work by a wide range of mechanisms.**
SEROTONIN ANTAGONISTS Granisetron hydrochloride (Kytril) Dolasetron mesylate (Anzemet) Ondansetron hydrochloride (Zofran) Palonestron (Aloxi)	**Serotonin antagonists suppress serotonin activity in the brain to prevent triggering of the vomiting reflex.**
Substance P/neurokinin (NK$_1$) receptor antagonist Aprepitant (Emend) Merck	Substance P/NK$_1$ receptor antagonists block nausea and vomiting pathways. They are given with a serotonin antagonist and dexamethasone to prevent nausea and vomiting.

*Drug information has been drawn from *The Physicians' Desk Reference*, the FDA web site, CancerSource.com Drug Guide, and, in some cases, specific pharmaceutical companies' web sites. Not all known side effects are listed here; consult with your doctor if you are experiencing side effects, whether they are listed here or not. Many of these medications also have interactions with other medications that produce symptoms not listed here.

ed if these fail or are used in combination with hormonal therapies. The side effects listed in Table 4 don't always occur—they vary depending on the individual, the dose, and other factors. However, any side effects that do occur, including some that may not be on this list, should be discussed with your doctor (see Question 49).

There has been much progress in the treatment of women with early breast cancer, as well as for those women with advanced disease. One such advance in the adjuvant treatment of early breast cancer is dose dense

Treatment

chemotherapy. Dose-dense chemotherapy is given more frequently (treatments every 2 weeks instead of 3), which allows higher doses to be given; studies have shown women undergoing this treatment have a lower risk of cancer recurring.

Studies are being conducted to determine the best treatment for women who are "triple negative" (that is, ER/PR negative and HER2 negative) as this subtype of breast cancer may be more difficult to treat. Scientists have been able to identify 21 genes that help determine whether a woman is likely to have her cancer recur. As this test (Oncotype DX) becomes more widely available, it will help women with early breast cancer and their doctors know whether they should get adjuvant treatment. For women with recurrent breast cancer, new agents are available, such as gemcitabine and Paclitaxel protein-bound particles for injectable suspension, nanoparticle albumin-bound (nab) paclitaxel (Abraxane). This new paclitaxel formulation is protein bound, so it allows higher drug doses to be given and more of the drug paclitaxel to enter the cancer cells.

Adjuncts

a variety of drugs that complement the chemotherapy regimen.

There is also a variety of drugs called **adjuncts** that complement the chemotherapy regimen. Although these technically are not chemotherapy drugs because they don't attack the cancer itself, they are part of the treatment because they alleviate complications of either the cancer or the treatment—biologic agents that promote white blood cell growth, for example. Some, such as leucovorin (a derivative of the vitamin folic acid), are used to enhance the performance of chemotherapy drugs. In the case of leucovorin, it enhances the performance of 5-FU but can also offset the side effects of methotrexate, so all three are commonly used in combination. Other adjuncts are used to combat conditions that sometimes occur in tandem with breast cancer. Among the most common complications, as mentioned in Question 35, are bone metastasis and hypercalcemia (accelerated loss of calcium in the bones accompanied by elevated levels of calcium in the bloodstream). This condition can create pain in the bones as well as heighten the risk of fractures and breaks, particularly among older women. The standard treatment for this condition is a bisphosphonate, either pamidronate or zoledronic acid (see Table 4).

49. I've heard dreadful stories about chemotherapy. What are some of the side effects, and how can they be alleviated?

Chemotherapy has many side effects; some of the most common ones are listed in Table 4. The drugs used in chemotherapy generally target frequently dividing cells; therefore, hair, bone marrow, and the mucous membranes lining the mouth, nose, and gastrointestinal tract are usually affected most. Even though side effects are common during chemotherapy, patients should let the caregiver know how the sessions are making them feel, because many side effects can be treated.

Hair loss (alopecia) is among the best known of the common side effects, which also include nausea, vomiting, hot flashes, mouth sores, and weight gain. A more serious (but less obvious) side effect that occurs commonly is decreased counts of various types of blood cells. This problem occurs because the chemotherapy kills bone marrow cells, which are necessary for production of blood cells. Although these side effects are invisible, they have significant impact on the patient's well-being; for example, decreases in white cells can increase the patient's susceptibility to infections, so it's important that patients on chemotherapy protect themselves from catching colds or infections. A decrease in the number of platelets can prevent blood from clotting, so similar precautions against cuts and injuries are likewise important. If the cancer chemotherapy lowers the blood count too much, then growth factors may be given to protect against infection and help the recovery of the cells (white and red blood cells). As with other types of cancer treatment, the type and severity of side effects vary depending on which drugs are given, as well as the patient's overall health. Additionally, after chemotherapy treatments are over, most side effects subside, and hair grows back.

Many side effects can be treated.

In premenopausal women, chemotherapy drugs can cause menstrual periods to halt, either temporarily or permanently, although such premature menopause is not common. However, the absence of menstruation does not necessarily mean you cannot get pregnant while on chemotherapy; it's not common, but it does happen. Because chemotherapy is toxic to dividing cells, it's extremely important that you take precautions against pregnancy during chemotherapy, because should you become pregnant while on chemo, the drugs will likely cause birth defects. If you are already pregnant when your cancer is diagnosed, it is vital to the health of your child that you let your doctor know as soon as possible so he or she can choose the treatment regimen least likely to harm the fetus; depending on the stage of fetal development, some chemotherapy regimens can still be used without risking birth defects. See Questions 93 and 94 for more discussion of breast cancer and pregnancy.

With all chemotherapy regimens, you will receive written information about possible side effects, and you may be asked to sign a consent form acknowledging that you have been given this information, have discussed it with your doctor, and wish to go ahead with treatment. When you fill out this paperwork, don't hesitate to ask questions about the effect of these drugs on your body—you shouldn't sign the forms until you are confident that you know what to expect. Individual drugs can have other side effects, which fortunately are not common but are more severe than the ones listed in the table. Your doctor will monitor you for signs of these side effects and change your treatment should you show symptoms of them. It is extremely important that you let your doctor or nurse know of any changes in your physical condition during chemotherapy so he or she can accurately assess your condition.

The National Cancer Institute offers booklets on chemotherapy, available both in printed form and online (see the appendix). There are also numerous online guides that discuss chemotherapy; many, including the American Cancer Society, even provide a database describing drugs used in cancer treatment, where you can search for your prescriptions and find highly specific information. These and similar guides are worth looking at to get a detailed idea of what you might expect from chemotherapy.

Popular wisdom about chemotherapy is that patients who go through it suffer from severe nausea and vomiting, hair loss, pain, and tiredness. There is some truth to this picture: nausea and vomiting, alopecia, pain, and fatigue are common side effects of some chemotherapy regimens, and for some women, particularly those with advanced cancer, these side effects can be debilitating. Nevertheless, the extent of these symptoms has been greatly overemphasized, which is unfortunate because it makes many patients hesitant to agree to a course of treatment that could lengthen or save their lives. Yes, some patients do find chemotherapy difficult, but keep

Treatment

When you consider that the end result could mean ridding your body of cancer altogether, it's worth running the risk of feeling awful for a few weeks or months.

in mind the learned response from previous experiences with vomiting; anticipating that nausea and vomiting will occur as it did previously triggers the actual reflex. It is important to remember that most patients do not experience such severe reactions to chemotherapy drugs, and a few have no reaction at all. And when you consider that the end result could mean ridding your body of cancer altogether, it's worth running the risk of feeling awful for a few days every three weeks or so.

Nausea/vomiting

Nausea and vomiting is not a topic most people care to discuss, but it's something that cancer patients must learn to deal with—these symptoms occur in almost 50% of patients undergoing chemotherapy and radiation therapy for cancer. The best way to approach the problem is to understand it, and this means knowing how to classify the symptoms. The National Comprehensive Cancer Network publishes patient guidelines (see the appendix) that detail five different classes of nausea and vomiting: acute-onset, delayed-onset, anticipatory, breakthrough, and refractory. **Acute-onset nausea and vomiting** usually occur a few minutes to several hours after the chemotherapy is given, with the worst episodes occurring 5 or 6 hours after treatment; the symptoms end within the first 24 hours. **Delayed-onset vomiting** develops more than 24 hours after chemotherapy is given. It occurs commonly with cisplatin, carboplatin, cyclophosphamide, and doxorubicin, but the timing and duration depends on the particular drug. **Anticipatory nausea and vomiting** are learned from previous experiences with vomiting. As the patient prepares for the next dose of chemotherapy, she anticipates that nausea and vomiting will occur as it did previously, which triggers the actual reflex. **Breakthrough vomiting** occurs despite treatment

Acute-onset nausea and vomiting

usually occur a few minutes to several hours after the chemotherapy is given.

Delayed-onset vomiting

develops more than 24 hours after chemotherapy is given.

Anticipatory nausea and vomiting

learned from previous experiences with vomiting; anticipating that nausea and vomiting will occur as it did previously triggers the actual reflex.

Breakthrough vomiting

occurs despite treatment to prevent it and requires additional therapy.

Refractory vomiting

antinausea treatments no longer induce any response in the patient.

to prevent it and requires additional therapy, while **refractory vomiting** occurs after one or more chemotherapy treatments—essentially if the patient is no longer responding to antinausea treatments.

Depending on the type of symptoms involved, different drugs called **antiemetics** are usually prescribed. Some common ones are listed in Table 4; all of these are examples of a class of drugs called serotonin antagonists that act upon the centers in the brain that trigger feelings of nausea. Antiemetic drugs are usually taken before the chemotherapy is given and/or at specific times related to when you take your chemotherapy pills, so it's important to be aware of the timing of your next treatment. In addition, some alternative techniques, including acupuncture and similar methods, are effective in controlling nausea (see Question 55). With the development of new antiemetics, it is possible to prevent nausea and vomiting. It is very important to tell your nurse or doctor if you have nausea and/or vomiting. The anti-metic regimen can be changed so that you do not get sick after the next cycle of chemotherapy.

There are other things you can do in your daily life to limit these symptoms. The Royal Marsden Hospital, a leading cancer center in England, advises its patients as described in Table 5.

Hair loss

Hair loss is a common side effect of chemotherapy. Although it is not physically painful or life threatening, it can cause great distress among women because loss of their hair makes them feel as though they're losing their beauty and sexual attraction. It is important to get a wig before you start losing your hair, as this will make

Antiemetics
antinausea medications.

Treatment

Table 5   Eating and Drinking to Avoid Nausea

- If you're feeling sick, you may find it helps to take a short walk before a meal and to eat in a room with good ventilation. Wear loose, comfortable clothing. Take an antiemetic half an hour before you eat.

- If you have been vomiting, you may find that this is the best time to try eating. Sucking an antacid tablet may prevent the acidic burning sensation that follows vomiting.

- If you are not keeping any food down for long periods of time, you should discuss this with your doctor, as you may need to be given some essential supplements.

- It's more important to drink plenty of liquid than to have three meals a day. Try sipping clear, cold fluids, such as water and soft drinks, slowly through a straw. Fizzy drinks like soda water and ginger ale are quite refreshing.

- Lemon, peppermint, or ginger teas have a pleasant taste and are also refreshing. The last two may also help to relieve nausea. It may help to avoid coffee, which has a strong taste and may also make you thirstier. Avoid alcohol as this can cause dehydration.

- You may find sucking ice cubes helps to freshen your mouth. These can be flavored with cordial or fruit juice. Crushed ice may make a drink more enjoyable. Some people find sucking lemon-flavoured sweets or mints reduces nausea.

- You may need to change your meal times and have small, frequent meals or snacks. Eat slowly and chew your food well. After a meal, relax in a sitting or slightly reclined position, instead of lying down. You may find it helps to eat light meals on the day of your chemotherapy. Don't eat for one or two hours before or after your treatment.

- Cold food or food served at room temperature, such as a sandwich, is usually less likely to upset you. Also, avoid very sweet, spicy, or greasy foods. Stay with bland foods, such as cereals, bread, or plain biscuits (crackers). Dry toast or ginger-nut biscuits may help settle your stomach.

- Try to breathe through your mouth because food smells often make nausea worse. Avoid foods with a strong smell. When you feel nauseated, ask friends or relatives to help prepare and serve food.

Adapted with permission from the Royal Marsden Hospital, Patient Information—Coping with Nausea and Vomiting (2001). (www.royalmarsden.org).

coping with hair loss a lot easier. Hair loss usually begins about a week and a half to three weeks after treatment starts and generally ends in complete hairlessness all over the body. When you lose your hair, you need to remember that the scalp will be extremely sensitive—it's not accustomed to being unprotected. You'll need to take extra steps to protect the skin of your head from sunlight or harsh clothing, such as wool hats, until your hair grows back. The good news is that it generally *will* grow back, just as thick and healthy as it was when you started, although it might change in texture; in most women, hair begins to grow back immediately once treatment has ended, and some even start to get their hair back while chemotherapy is still ongoing.

At the moment, there's no treatment for hair loss. Some researchers are investigating topical drugs to prevent hair loss. At this time, some experimental treatments show promise, but are not ready for clinical trials. See Question 59 for more information on dealing with hair loss.

Pain

Pain is another common side effect of cancer treatment, and it occurs with all three forms (surgery, radiation, and chemotherapy). Surgery is accompanied by pain because cutting into or around nerve tissue damages it, particularly if you have had extensive lymph node dissection, and pain is the body's way of alerting you to that injury. As nerve endings regenerate or inflammation decreases, the pain usually subsides. With radiation and chemotherapy, the pain usually consists of dull, achy discomfort, but it can also flair up into very severe episodes of pain. Treating pain with strong medications can have its own complications: some pain drugs can cause drowsiness, confusion, constipation, or other uncomfortable side effects, and some particularly strong medications can be addictive if misused. However, the fear of these complications is generally exaggerated, which obstructs effective pain management, so it's important that you have an accurate sense of how your pain should be dealt with. See Questions 57 and 58 for more information about controlling pain.

Fatigue

Fatigue is a normal reaction to the strain of rebuilding damaged cells.

Cancer patients often experience fatigue. It is the most common side effect of chemotherapy, as well as radiation therapy. It is a complicated side effect because there are many factors that contribute to feelings of tiredness. Sometimes, as shown in Table 4, it is a side effect of the chemotherapy drugs. It's also a common side effect of radiation therapy. It can even occur spontaneously in the absence of either of these adjuvant therapies. Yet resting—which seems the obvious solution for fatigue—sometimes does more harm than good: rest too much, and your energy level actually decreases. So how is fatigue properly dealt with?

Unlike most other symptoms, fatigue is the one side effect that often isn't treated medically, but through adjustments in diet and lifestyle. The reason for this is simple: fatigue is a symptom that comes and goes, that isn't predictable in onset or duration, and usually reflects the exertion of the body as it attempts to heal. Unlike nausea or hair loss, fatigue isn't a sign of bodily *dys*function except when it's related to low blood cell counts; it's a normal reaction to the strain of rebuilding damaged cells, healing injuries, and fighting off illness, all of which are going on during the time a patient is undergoing treatment. As you undergo treatment, all of the healing systems of your body are pushing ahead full power to heal the damage being done by both the cancer and the treatment; the fatigue you feel is your body's way of signaling that you need rest and good nutrition to support this effort. "Curing" fatigue through the use of stimulants would simply wear out the body more in the long term, leaving it more vulnerable to opportunistic infections. Thus, except where red blood cell counts have dropped—something your doctor will monitor throughout your treatment—fatigue is not a symptom to be treated with medication, but is rather a signal that you should find ways to "reassign" your body's energy stores. Question 50 addresses some methods of handling fatigue; other resources offering solutions can be found in the appendix.

There are many other side effects, too many to list here—we've mentioned only the four most common, and, in this respect, barely touched the surface. For more information on managing side effects, you can check any of the resources listed in the appendix. Side effects and quality of life are among the most important issues facing cancer patients, so there are many resources addressing these problems. More discussion of specific quality-of-life issues will follow.

50. What can I do about fatigue? Why do I have more energy some days, less on others?

Fatigue need not rule your life; you simply need to learn how to budget your energy to accomplish the necessary tasks of day-to-day life. It may take you a few weeks to figure out how to pace yourself, but once you learn how much energy you have from day to day, you can adjust your activities to accommodate the limits set by the healing process. The confusing thing about fatigue is that it's not constant from one day to the next. Some days, you'll feel completely wrung out, to the point that even breathing seems tiring. Other days, you'll feel as good as you ever did before your diagnosis. Still others, you'll feel lousy all morning—but the minute you walk into the doctor's office for your check-up, you suddenly feel fine. Part of the reason for these strange swings in energy levels is the action of **adrenaline**: when you are suddenly faced with an important or stressful event, such as a doctor's visit, your body responds with this hormone to prepare your body for "fight or flight" reactions. It doesn't matter whether the event is good or bad—any sort of excitement will cause the reaction in your body, and you'll pay for the adrenaline rush later with muscle weakness and fatigue. These abrupt swings in energy are perfectly normal, but can be very frustrating in their unpredictability.

As noted above, rest and sleep are very important— your bodily systems are working vigorously and require a recharge period—but get too much, and it will backfire: you'll feel more tired, not less. This effect is called **deconditioning**; as you spend more time in bed, you retain less water in the body, which causes fatigue, weakness, and dizziness. The heart and cardiovascular system are most affected by this problem, and you may find yourself feeling dizzy and breathless when you get up after a long period of bed rest. Clearly, if you've already begun to experience deconditioning, you won't be able to abruptly swing into the kind of activity that would recondition you, but if you move from your bed to a chair, drink plenty of fluids, and perform mild activities that keep you moving—knitting, grooming a pet, or slow, gentle, in-chair exercises—you can start to counteract the deconditioning effects.

Adrenaline

a hormone triggered by an important or stressful event that prepares the body for "fight or flight" reactions.

Deconditioning

fatigue, weakness, and dizziness caused by spending too much time at rest and asleep.

Nutrition is another key to combating fatigue, particularly when the problem is connected to low counts of red blood cells (**anemia**). Your doctor will monitor your blood counts and may have you consult with a dietitian if you need advice on how to offset fatigue with nutrition. But don't start taking dietary or herbal supplements without alerting your doctor first—even common supplements might have interactions with your ongoing treatment (see Question 55 for more on supplements). The nutritionist assigned to your team will give you a number of tips for getting the best possible nutrition during your treatment. This may mean changing your diet substantially—many Americans eat a less-than-ideal diet and don't even realize it—but don't turn it into a self-denial situation. This "diet" is not a weight-loss regimen—quite the opposite. If you find that certain "unhealthy" foods seem appealing, go ahead and eat them; just try to balance the nonnutritious items with fruits, vegetables, and other foods your nutritionist will recommend. Bear in mind the types of foods that could trigger nausea, as listed in Question 49, and try to avoid them; concentrate instead on foods that supply plenty of vitamins and minerals—fruits and vegetables particularly—and complex carbohydrates, such as whole wheat breads or crackers. Refer to the food pyramid (see http://www.fda.gov) as a guideline when shopping to make sure you have a variety of the foods you need for a balanced diet on hand. Always remember to drink plenty of fluids, and avoid caffeine, alcohol, and greasy or spicy foods. If nausea or diarrhea becomes a problem, fall back on the BRAT system—bananas, plain rice, apples or applesauce, and dry toast, all foods that soothe an upset gastrointestinal tract while providing necessary nutrients. There are many resources available to help you plan your diet; see the appendix for a list.

Anemia

a low count of red blood cells.

Treatment

Conserve your energy whenever possible by spreading your activities throughout the day and taking frequent rest breaks. Do as many tasks as possible while seated; try to obtain a lightweight folding chair to carry with you when you run errands or go to the grocery store, because it will enable you to sit down and rest should fatigue strike unexpectedly while you're out and about. Find "energy restoratives"—activities that you enjoy that don't require much physical effort, such as listening to music, reading, bird watching, or looking at pictures. Ask friends or family members to take on certain high-energy tasks for you, such as housework, laundry, or childcare.

As you grow accustomed to the limits of your energy levels, you'll be able to avoid wild swings in energy from one day to the next. However, if you have trouble sleeping or find yourself in a state of severe, constant fatigue, consult with members of your team, particularly your nutritionist and your oncology nurse; they will be best able to advise you. For other resources on beating fatigue, see the appendix.

51. What is a clinical trial? Should I consider joining a clinical trial?

There are several different types of clinical trials. Some are aimed at finding better ways to screen for and prevent cancer, while others look at potential new treatments, and still others study ways to improve the quality of life for cancer patients. For this discussion, only treatment trials are relevant.

Treatment trials are run to test the effectiveness of new treatments, whether they are newly developed cancer drugs, new combinations of known drugs, new approaches to surgery or radiation therapy, or even new classes of therapy altogether, such as gene therapy. Although such trials are usually conducted either by independent research laboratories associated with universities or hospitals or by the research branches of drug companies, oversight of the process is controlled by the Food and Drug Administration (FDA) of the U.S. government. The treatment usually will have been tested in laboratory animals to see how the animals respond prior to testing in humans; this weeds out the treatments likely to prove too dangerous or toxic to be useful. The human tests proceed in a series of steps called **phases**. The results from each phase must be reviewed by the FDA before the laboratory developing the drug is permitted to move into the next phase.

Phases

a series of steps followed in clinical trials.

In Phase I trials, a drug that was shown to be effective in studies with animals is tried for the first time in humans. Generally, these studies enroll only small numbers of patients and are focused on two questions: first, what technique is best for administering the drug, and second, what dose of the drug is effective without creating intolerable side effects in humans.

If the drug shows good results in Phase I, it will move next to Phase II trials, which continue this process with larger numbers of patients. Phase II trials refine the tests to determine how well the drug works and in which types of cancer the drug works best.

Phase III trials test a drug against the current standard of care. After all, even if the drug is effective, it doesn't make much sense to continue developing it if it is less effective and has greater side effects than a drug currently in use. These trials usually include a very large population of patients and are sometimes conducted through clinics and doctors' offices that agree to participate. If the drug passes this phase of testing, it is submitted to the FDA for final review and approval.

There are a number of good reasons for considering participating in a clinical trial. For one thing, if you do participate, you'll be cared for by physicians who are familiar with the very latest information about cancer treatment, and your condition will be monitored very closely. If the drug or procedure being tested is beneficial, you could be one of the first people to benefit from it—and your participation could make it possible for this drug to reach a wider range of people with breast cancer who would not have it if volunteers like you didn't participate in these trials. Particularly if you aren't responding well to approved therapies, a clinical trial could give you an alternative that will work better than the drugs currently on the market.

But there are drawbacks too. New drugs and procedures may have side effects or risks unknown to the doctors, or be less effective than current approaches. Even if a drug or procedure does work well, it may not work well for *you*; not all patients respond the same way to the same treatments, and the goal of these trials is to find something that works for *most* people, not *all* people. There is a possibility that the treatment will leave you in worse condition, not better. Also, there's no guarantee that you'll actually *get* the new treatment, because most trials compare a group of experimental patients receiving the new treatment to a group of similar people, called "controls," who receive either **placebos** (sugar pills) or standard therapies. You will be required to make more visits to the doctor so he or she can closely monitor your progress, and any deviation from the regimen could

Placebos
sugar pills.

mean you're excluded from the trial. So in some ways, joining a clinical trial may make your day-to-day life more difficult; only you can decide whether these problems are worth the potential benefits.

Any decision to participate in clinical trials should be discussed with your doctor prior to joining. Take the time to research the available trials through Internet searches (NCI's CancerTrials service is a good place to start) or library research. Most trials' results are published in medical journals, so a search of Phase I or Phase II trials of drugs used in treating your cancer could lead you to a Phase III trial just under way. If you do find a trial that seems suitable, make sure you thoroughly review its **protocol**—the research plan for how the drug is given and to whom it is given—to make sure you fit the profile of patients being included in testing; for example, if the protocol is designed for premenopausal women and you're over 70, you will not be eligible. If you apply for and are accepted into a trial, you'll be asked to review and sign an **informed consent** form that will give you all the necessary information about what you'll be testing, what known effects it has, and what possible benefits (or harm) it could do. Don't just sign it right away; take the time to read it carefully, discuss it with your doctor and family members, and ask the research team all of the questions that occur to you, no matter how trivial or silly you might think they are. A clinical trial is not something to take lightly, and the researchers need to know that you thoroughly understand what you're getting yourself into. Remember, too, that even if you enroll in a clinical trial, you always have the right to withdraw or stop at any time.

Protocol

the research plan for how the drug is given and to whom it is given.

Informed consent

a process by which patients participating in a clinical study are provided with all available information regarding the experimental treatment prior to consenting to receive that treatment.

52. What is meant by hormonal therapy?

Questions 9 and 47 discuss the fact that some cancers grow faster in the presence of the hormones estrogen and progesterone. As previously mentioned, lab tests can determine which hormones, if any, make a tumor grow more rapidly; cancers that respond to estrogen are categorized as ER+ and those that respond to progesterone are described as PR+. Some cancers respond to both (ER+/PR+), others don't respond to either one (ER-/PR-). Finding out your tumor's ER and PR status will be one of the first steps your oncologist takes so that he or she can determine the best strategy for treating your cancer. In Question 47, we described how hormonal therapy works on such cancers, but it's worth briefly repeating that discussion here. Unlike standard chemotherapy, which targets all fast-growing cells in the body indiscriminately, hormonal or endocrine therapy is tailored specifically toward those tumors that respond to the presence of estrogen or progesterone. The agents used in hormone therapy (described in Table 6) block the action of these hormones so they can't encourage growth in cancer cells. This is important because even when a surgeon has removed a tumor and the original site of the tumor has been treated with radiation to kill any remaining tumor cells, there is no guarantee that a few cancerous cells didn't escape. Hormone therapy can prevent such cells from growing and establishing new tumors elsewhere, either within the remaining breast tissue or as metastatic tumors in other parts of the body

There are several types of drugs used to accomplish these goals. The most common way to suppress the body's production of hormones is through two classes of drugs: antihormones and **aromatase inhibitors** (see Table 6). The antihormones class currently consists of one

(continued on page 139)

Table 6   Hormonal Therapies Used in Breast Cancer Treatment

Drug Name Generic (Brand), Maker	Type/Effects	Used For:
Anastrozole (Arimidex) AstraZeneca Pharmaceuticals	Aromatase inhibitor (reversible); prevents production of estrogen in adrenal glands	Initial adjuvant treatment of post-menopausal women with hormone receptor–positive breast cancer.
Exemestane (Aromasin) Pfizer	Aromatase inhibitor (irreversible)	Adjuvant treatment of advanced breast cancer in postmenopausal women who have received 2–3 years of tamoxifen and are switched to exemestane to complete the 5 years of tamoxifen therapy.
Fulvestrant injection (Faslodex) AstraZeneca Pharmaceuticals	Estrogen receptor antagonist	Treatment of hormone receptor–positive metastatic breast cancer in postmenopausal women whose disease has progressed after anti-estrogen therapy.
Letrozole (Femara) Novartis Pharmaceuticals	Aromatase inhibitor (reversible)	Adjuvant treatment of postmenopausal women with hormone receptor positive early breast cancer. The effectiveness of Femara in early breast cancer is based on an analysis of disease-free survival in patients treated for a median of 24 months and followed for a median of 26 months. Follow up analyses will determine long-term outcomes for both safety and efficacy. Femara is also used for the extended adjuvant treatment of early breast cancer in postmenopausal women who have received 5 years of adjuvant tamoxifen therapy. The effectiveness of Femara in extended adjuvant treatment of early breast cancer is based on an analysis of disease-free survival in patients treated for a median of 24 months. Further data will be required to determine long-term outcome. Femara is also used for first-line treatment of post-menopausal women with hormone receptor positive or hormone receptor unknown locally advanced or metastatic breast cancer. Femara is also indicated for the treatment of advanced breast cancer in postmenopausal women with disease progression following antiestrogen therapy.
Megestrol acetate (Megace) Bristol-Myers Squibb	Aromatase inhibitor; mimics action of progesterone, blocking it from progesterone receptors	Used to treat PR+ cancers. Because it is also an appetite stimulant, may be preferred for underweight patients who have responsive cancers.

continues

Table 6 *continued*

Drug Name		
Generic (Brand), Maker	Type/Effects	Used For:
Tamoxifen citrate (Nolvadex) AstraZeneca Pharmaceuticals	Binds to estrogen receptors, blocking estrogen from the cancer cells	NOLVADEX is effective in the treatment of metastatic breast cancer in women and men. In premenopausal women with metastatic breast cancer, NOLVADEX is an alternative to oophorectomy or ovarian irradiation. Available evidence indicated that patients whose tumors are estrogen receptor positive are more likely to benefit from NOLVADEX therapy. **Adjuvant Treatment of Breast Cancer:** NOLVADEX is indicated for the treatment of node-positive breast cancer in postmenopausal women following total mastectomy or segmental mastectomy, axillary dissection, and breast irradiation. NOLVADEX is also indicated for the treatment of axillary node-negative breast cancer in women following total mastectomy or segmental mastectomy, axillary dissection, and breast irradiation. In addition, NOLVADEX reduces the occurrence of contralateral breast cancer in patients receiving adjuvant therapy with NOLVADEX for breast cancer. **Ductal Carcinoma in Situ (DCIS):** In women with DCIS, following breast surgery and radiation, NOLVADEX is indicated to reduce the risk of invasive breast cancer. (See **BOXED WARNING** at the beginning of full Prescribing Information.) **Reduction in Breast Cancer Incidence in High Risk Women:** NOLVADEX is indicated to reduce the incidence of breast cancer in women at high risk for breast cancer. NOLVADEX is indicated only for high-risk women. "High risk" is defined as women at least 35 years of age with a 5-year predicted risk of breast cancer $\geq 1.67\%$, as calculated by the Gail Model. (See **BOXED WARNING** at the beginning of enclosed full Prescribing Information.)
Toremifene citrate (Fareston) Orion Corporation	Aromatase inhibitor	Treatment of metastatic breast cancer in postmenopausal women with ER+ or receptor–unknown tumors.

approved drug, tamoxifen, which is widely prescribed and often used as the first step in hormonal therapy (see Question 53 on tamoxifen). Because of concerns regarding tamoxifen's effect on the uterus, a second antihormone, raloxifene, is currently being studied, but it has not yet reached the stage at which it can be approved by the FDA for this use. Aromatase inhibitors suppress an enzyme called aromatase that is essential to production of estrogen, thus reducing the amount of estrogen available to promote tumor growth. In the past, tamoxifen therapy was always tried first, and aromatase inhibitors have been the second line of defense. While tamoxifen blocks the estrogen receptor in breast tumors that are positive for this receptor, new data indicates that aromatase inhibitors (AIs), such as anastrozole (Arimidex), can be used initially instead of tamoxifen, since the studies showed AIs were superior in post menopausal women. AIs, such as letrozole (Femara), or exemestane (Aromasin), may be started in postmenopausal women who have been receiving tamoxifen for two to five years. Once an AI is started, the use may be continued for up to five years. AIs are replacing tamoxifen as the most widely used hormone treatment for breast cancer. In addition, AIs differ slightly—studies show that when a woman stops responding to one AI, another may be just as effective. Studies are looking at the best sequence to use the different AIs, tamoxifen, and fulvestrant. AIs have less side effects than tamoxifen, which can cause endometrial cancer and blood clots. However, because AIs do such a good job blocking estrogen, they can cause osteoporosis and increased risk of fractures. Studies continue to be done to see which drug, and for how long, is best for different types of women. Chemotherapy also lowers the level of estrogen in the blood of many premenopausal women.

Whichever method is used, the goal is the same: to starve the cancerous cells of the estrogen they need to keep growing. If this goal is accomplished, the cancer cells die, and the tumor's growth slows or even stops. This can be of benefit before surgery in patients with fast-growing cancers that are not able to have surgery right away for one reason or another, but hormonal therapy is more commonly used as a means of starving any remaining cancer cells to prevent recurrence in patients whose tumor has already been removed. It can also be used to limit the growth of tumors in a patient whose cancer has already metastasized, particularly if the metastasis is in a location that isn't easily treated by surgery or radiation, such as the bones or the liver.

Another type of hormonal therapy includes fulvestrant (Faslodex) which was approved by the FDA in April 2002, for treatment of postmenopausal women with hormone receptor positive metastatic breast cancer. This drug is classified as an **estrogen-receptor antagonist**. Unlike the aromatase inhibitors or antihormones, which either suppress the body's hormone production or block the hormones before they can bind to receptors in the tumor, fulvestrant attacks the tumor's estrogen receptors, damaging them so that they are unable to bind to estrogen. This difference is significant because some patients become resistant to other forms of hormonal therapy. It permits an alternative approach to advanced cancers that no longer respond to traditional hormone therapy. Clinical trials are currently testing it against, and in combination with, the aromatase inhibitor anastrozole and against tamoxifen after AI failure to determine which therapy is most effective.

Estrogen-receptor antagonist
drug that attacks a tumor's estrogen receptors, damaging them so that they are unable to bind to estrogen.

OTHER THERAPIES

53. I had a radical mastectomy years ago, and my doctor says I should take tamoxifen now. What is it? Are there any side effects with tamoxifen?

Tamoxifen is the most widely prescribed hormonal therapy treatment for early and advanced stage breast cancer. It has been used for more than 30 years to treat patients with advanced stage breast cancer, both as treatment to slow or stop tumor growth, and as a secondary or adjuvant therapy that prevents recurrence. Tamoxifen has shown considerable effectiveness in preventing recurrent cancer. Among participants in the Breast Cancer Prevention Trial funded by the National Cancer Institute, use of tamoxifen resulted in a nearly 50% decrease in diagnoses of both invasive and noninvasive breast cancer among high-risk women. Someone who has already had cancer would fall into this category of high-risk women, and a woman who had cancer 20 years ago, prior to the use of tamoxifen in cancer therapy, is at even greater risk because of her advancing age. The benefits of tamoxifen to post-menopausal, high-risk women are numerous, yet the use of this drug should be considered in the context of an individual's circumstances. Women with a family history of clotting disorders leading to stroke or heart attacks, for example, probably would be ill-advised to take tamoxifen as a prophylactic. Studies are being conducted to see how effective aromatase inhibitors (AIs) are in preventing breast cancer. Since AIs are more effective than tamoxifen in treating cancer and preventing it from coming back, it is hoped AIs will be more effective in prevention as well. Your risk of recurrent cancer versus risk from other health factors should be discussed with your doctor before deciding to take tamoxifen as preventive medicine.

Even though the AIs have been shown superior to ta-moxifen in the adjuvant setting (as additional treatment for early-stage disease after breast cancer is removed by surgery), tamoxifen shows encouraging results in prevent-ing cancer in women known to have very high risk (most have either the BCRA1 or BCRA2 mutation). This ap-plication of the drug is one of its most exciting aspects, but tamoxifen, like any systemic therapy, affects tissues other than the breast tissues for which it's prescribed, and some of its effects are not good. Studies have shown that there is some increased risk for cancer of the uterus, for example. In a small percentage of patients who take ta-moxifen along with chemotherapy, venous blood clots have been reported. These risks, however, are often much lower than the benefits received from tamoxifen, which—aside from its cancer-fighting properties—also lowers blood cholesterol and slows osteoporosis, benefits that are particularly important for postmenopausal women. The National Cancer Institute notes, "The benefits of tamox-ifen as a treatment for breast cancer are firmly established and far outweigh the potential risks." If you are prescribed tamoxifen, whether for cancer treatment or as a prophy-lactic, talk to your oncologist about any concerns you may have, and be sure your gynecologist and primary care doc-tor know that you're taking the drug so they'll be alert to the warning signs of either uterine cancer or clotting problems. You should have regular pelvic exams and noti-fy your doctor about any unusual bleeding or pain.

54. What is meant by adjuvant therapy? Is it the same as alternative therapy?

Adjuvant therapy is treatment given after the primary treatment to increase the chances of a cure. With breast cancer, the primary treatment is usually surgery, sometimes combined with radiation; adjuvant therapy may include chemotherapy, radiation therapy, or hormone therapy. Sometimes, adjuvant therapy is started before the primary treatment; this is called **neoadjuvant therapy**, but its purpose is still the same: it's used to supplement the primary treatment to increase the chances of a cure. The type of adjuvant therapy selected depends on the stage and type of cancer. Adjuvant and neoadjuvant therapies are nearly always composed of standard drugs or treatments.

For the purpose of this discussion, we'll use "therapy" to refer only to those treatments that make use of a substance to make physiological alterations in the body; mental techniques, such as imaging, meditation, and prayer, will be considered later, in Questions 55 and 60. **Alternative therapy** (medicines used in lieu of standard medical therapies) and **complementary therapy** (medicines used in conjunction with standard therapies) include a variety of herbal and food remedies, vitamins and other supplements, and traditional treatments such as acupuncture. Such therapies have become increasingly popular with the general public, and many are based upon traditional healing practices that have hundreds of years of use. Whether they actually work depends on the therapy you pick. Some alternative therapies are nothing more than scams taking advantage of patients' fears and longings for *anything* that will make the illness go away. They may do no harm—although some herbal agents *can* harm you— but they also do no good, so you're spending your money for no good reason. However, some of these nonstandard remedies are effective, though not necessarily as effective as standard therapies. For more on alternative therapies, see Question 55.

Neoadjuvant therapy
adjuvant therapy that is started before the primary treatment.

Alternative therapy
medicines used in lieu of standard medical therapies.

Complementary therapy
medicines used in conjunction with standard therapies.

Treatment

55. Are there alternative or herbal treatments for breast cancer and its side effects? Do they work?

We may be most familiar with modern Western medicine, but many people are becoming increasingly aware of, and attracted to, alternative philosophies of patient care, particularly east and south Asian methods, homeopathic, and naturopathic medical systems. Though some people are skeptical of the effectiveness of these treatment methodologies, some of the herbs and techniques used in alternative systems have been shown to have legitimate healing properties. Yet there are so many medicines and therapies touted as the next new treatment for cancer, it's hard to know where to start: everything from shark cartilage to green tea extract to vitamin C to melatonin has been suggested as having curative properties. For a cancer patient anxious to find an effective treatment—or even a way to deal with unpleasant side effects—the list can be bewildering, yet a recent study of cancer patients showed that as many of 80% were using or had tried such treatments in conjunction with their standard therapeutic regimens, in the hope of either enhancing the action of the regimen or reducing the side effects caused by it. Unfortunately, a large proportion of the patients in the study were taking these alternative therapies without letting their doctors know and suffering side effects as the therapies interfered with or interacted with the action of chemotherapy drugs, which is why many physicians are wary of alternative medicines. Yet part of the problem is that doctors fail to ask whether their patients are using alternative therapies, and patients don't think to tell them. So the most important point to make in any discussion of alternative therapies is: *Make sure your doctor knows about them before you start using them.*

Traditional Asian medicine is attractive to many people because it emphasizes a whole-body approach to disease. From this perspective, disease is the product of improper balance or disturbances of vital energies that connect mind, body, spirit, and emotion. To treat such imbalances, traditional Oriental medicine uses techniques including acupuncture, herbal medicine, oriental massage, and qi gong, a technique based on controlled breathing and meditation.

Homeopathic and naturopathic medicine are also examples of complete alternative medical systems. Homeopathic medicine is an unconventional Western system that is based on the principle that "like cures like," that is, the same substance that in large doses produces the symptoms of an illness, in very minute doses cures it. Naturopathic medicine views disease as a sign that the processes by which the body naturally heals itself are out of balance and emphasizes health restoration rather than disease treatment. Naturopathic physicians employ an array of healing practices, including diet and clinical nutrition; homeopathy; acupuncture; herbal medicine; hydrotherapy (the use of water in a range of temperatures and methods of application); spinal and soft-tissue manipulation; physical therapies involving electric currents, ultrasound, and light therapy; therapeutic counseling; and pharmacology.

The list of alternative and complementary treatments is too long to discuss in depth, but there are a few treatments that have been shown to be effective in treating cancer symptoms and side effects; these will be discussed next. For more information on treatments not discussed here, visit the Web site of the National Institutes of Health's National Center for Complementary and Alternative Medicine, which hosts a clearinghouse of information on various alternative treatments (see the appendix).

Many people are becoming increasingly aware of, and attracted to, alternative philosophies of patient care.

Treatment

145

Acupuncture

There are some alternative therapies that have been shown to be effective against certain side effects, particularly nausea, fatigue, and pain. One of the best known is **acupuncture**, which is a Chinese therapy in use for over 2500 years involving the use of thin needles inserted into specific locations in the skin. In 1997, after studying the treatment at length, the National Institutes of Health concluded that acupuncture does provide substantial relief of nausea and vomiting associated with chemotherapy and that further research was necessary to determine whether it may have some benefits in treating pain associated with some forms of cancer therapy.

Acupuncture's effectiveness in controlling nausea has been well documented, and some insurance companies have even begun paying for acupuncture treatments. If you are interested in acupuncture as a therapy for nausea, consult with your doctor—he or she might have a list of approved practitioners in your area. If not, the American Academy of Medical Acupuncture (AAMA) keeps a list of accredited practitioners nationwide, as well as laws governing the practice for your state and information regarding how acupuncture should be used. Contact information for the AAMA can be found in the appendix.

Mind-body-spirit techniques

There are any number of techniques that focus the power of the mind and the spirit upon the body to help cure disease, including meditation, guided imagery, and prayer. These come in innumerable forms and can't be listed here, but the type of mind-body-spirit method a person might use is a very personal choice in any case. Do they work? That depends on what you expect of them. Studies have shown that mind-body-spirit techniques do affect practitioners in very positive ways, primarily with

Acupuncture

a Chinese therapy involving the use of thin needles inserted into specific locations in the skin.

respect to quality of life. They promote relaxation, a more positive outlook, and a general sense of well-being. And, as noted in Question 60, all of these feelings can promote increased immune activity, faster recovery, and better overall physiological health—but they work best in conjunction with standard treatments such as chemotherapy and radiation therapy. Most doctors would encourage their patients to make use of these techniques as adjuvant, not primary, treatments of cancer.

Herbal remedies and supplements

There are a number of herbal and supplemental treatments that are said to be effective for breast cancer, and still others that work on the side effects of standard treatment methods. Many of these have long histories of use in traditional societies, and, indeed, herbal and traditional medicines are often the source of medicinal compounds used in modern pharmaceuticals. Unfortunately, relatively few of even the best-known herbal remedies have undergone scientific testing to demonstrate their effectiveness. That doesn't mean they don't work—the few studies of herbal remedies that have been done show that some really do have positive effects. The basic problem, however, is that very few people, even trained herbalists with a genuine, legitimate knowledge of various herbs' pharmacologic properties, understand the full effects of these substances on the body—and there is extremely limited knowledge among herbalists and medical doctors alike of what interactions they might have with standard therapies. Worse still, ready availability of supplements allows patients to self-medicate with vitamins, supplements, and herbs they don't properly understand. Supplements currently are not regulated, or even reviewed, by the FDA, so there is no oversight of formulas used in different brands, the quantity of active ingredients, or the

Studies have shown that mind-body-spirit techniques do affect practitioners in very positive ways.

purity of those ingredients—in short, there's no guarantee that the bottle you buy from the health food store shelf contains what you think it does. Even if you try to make your own medicines with fresh ingredients, you could be asking for trouble if you don't have training in the preparation and use of herbs. This is not knowledge you can get from skimming through a book or looking on the Web: the correct use of herbs is a very tricky business, and in some cases, if you use too much or take it improperly (for example, eating it raw when you should be making a tea or infusion from its leaves) you can make yourself extremely sick, particularly if you're already taking chemotherapy drugs. Remember, during cancer treatment, your normal body systems are under extreme strain, and you could—with the best of intentions—overstrain your body if you take a supplement or herb without knowing its interactions and effects. *Never* begin a course of medication, of any type, without first checking with your doctor.

That said, some herbal medicines that have been studied show promising effects. For example, two common herbs—evening primrose and borage, commonly called starflower—have been used in Europe since the Middle Ages for treatment of premenstrual problems, including breast pain. Both contain a substance called gamma linolenic acid (GLA), an omega-6 fatty acid, which studies show can inhibit the spread of malignant tumors by restricting blood vessel growth. Phase I studies of GLA in England show that it enhances the effect of tamoxifen in some forms of breast cancer. Other common herbs and natural remedies address side effects such as nausea or depression. Ginger root, for example, is effective for treatment of nausea, while

St. John's Wort is an accepted natural remedy for mild depression. The latter, however, is also known to interact badly with some chemotherapy drugs, such as anthracyclines and etoposide. Other popular remedies for cancer, such as mistletoe, have been shown to have few effects in treating cancer, but there are herbs that stimulate responses in the immune system—echinacea, an extract of the purple coneflower, is among the best known of these—and others, such as garlic, that are natural antibiotics. Such herbs could be helpful in protecting the body against opportunistic infections while the immune system is overstressed by its battle against cancer. Yet both herbs have potential drawbacks: echinacea's stimulant effect works only in the short term, and long-term use can actually depress the immune system, while garlic can suppress blood clotting—a good thing, if you're at risk for stroke or clots, but a bad thing if you're about to undergo or are trying to heal from surgery. Thus, it's important to investigate herbal remedies thoroughly before taking them in conjunction with your treatment.

If you regularly use herbal preparations to treat minor illnesses, you don't necessarily have to abandon the practice—as noted above, they often do have beneficial effects. However, the stress of illness on your body is significant enough that you'd be well advised to consult with your doctor, your pharmacist, and a trained herbalist before using herbal medicines in conjunction with standard therapies. To find a trained herbalist, talk to the herbal specialist in your natural foods store or visit a store specializing in homeopathic medicine.

56. What happens if the treatment doesn't work? What happens if the cancer comes back?

Generally, if one treatment doesn't stop the cancer from growing, your medical team will switch to another—and if necessary, another, and another. Likewise, if cancer recurs, the team generally starts where it did with the original tumor—surgery, radiation, chemo—but may choose a different method of any or all of these treatments. For instance, if your initial tumor was treated with lumpectomy and external radiation, your recurrence might require mastectomy and chemotherapy. If chemotherapy drugs were used in your initial treatment, a more aggressive regimen might be called for the second time around. It all depends on how your recurrence presents itself.

Although advanced or recurrent cancer can be treated successfully with the standard arsenal of treatments, there is no hiding the fact that with every recurrence or advance in stage, the stakes become higher. After repeated cycles of cancer treatment, you might need to reconsider the goals of your treatment. Do you really want to continue going through chemotherapy and radiation with all the physical and emotional strains they place on you and your family in the hope of finally killing the cancer? Or would you prefer to switch to **palliative care**, care to relieve the symptoms of cancer and to keep the best quality of life for as long as possible?

Palliative care

care to relieve the symptoms of cancer and to keep the best quality of life for as long as possible without seeking to cure the cancer.

There are arguments to be made for both approaches. Some people feel that working toward anything short of an absolute cure is "giving up," and they will keep fighting as long as they can. This approach may ultimately result in a longer life, possibly even a cure—particularly since new approaches and drugs for treating advanced cancer are

150

being developed continually. So, just when some patients have reached the end of the line for conventional treatments, some new approach may appear on the horizon to extend their time. The downside is that you and your family and caregivers are under continuous strain throughout each cycle of treatments. Although there are ways to ease this strain (see Question 91), you can't get rid of it entirely.

Keeping up the fighting spirit can be draining for all of you. For some people, it's just not worth the effort—they'd rather accept the possibility of premature death, focusing instead upon having the best possible quality of life in whatever time is left to them. Sometimes, letting go of the worry about death can be an immense relief and can enrich your life and the lives of your loved ones. If death is a given, you can stop thinking about it and get on with day-to-day living—but, knowing your time is limited, you make the most of the days and let the small, petty concerns fall by the wayside.

Don't think you have to make this decision alone: talk to your family, a minister or counselor, and most especially, your health care team—it may be that they can find ways to help you alleviate some of the strain of treatment if you're growing tired of the fight. There are also ways for you to make sure you will be in control in the final phases of your illness. See Questions 67 and 68 for information on how to address end-of-life issues.

PART FIVE

Coping with Treatment and Side Effects

How can I relieve the pain associated with treatment?

More . . .

57. How can I relieve the pain associated with treatment?

How you handle pain depends on the type of pain it is, how severe it is, and how you feel about medication. Pain comes in two general varieties: severe, short-term or **acute pain**, and **chronic** or **persistent pain**, which can range in severity and is present for long periods of time, though not always at the same level of intensity. Occasionally, patients experience both types—a low-level chronic pain that can be kept under control may be interspersed with severe, acute pain that breaks through the treatment. Some forms of pain can be treated without resorting to drugs, which some patients find preferable due to side effects that can be associated with pain medication. Others require the use of pain killers of varying strengths.

Nonmedical Pain Relief

Have you ever had a cut or injury that didn't hurt until you actually saw the blood running from it? This situation isn't all that unusual. There's no physiological basis for it—your injury or illness isn't any worse than it was a minute ago, yet the moment you notice it, it feels a hundred times worse. Focusing your attention on pain gives a distinct perception that it hurts more. Pain-blocking techniques, including imaging (discussed further in Question 60), distraction, and hypnosis, all address the patient's perceptions of pain to give the patient a *perception* of relief—even though the physical source of the pain is still present and active, it really doesn't matter if the patient doesn't actually feel the pain. Most of these techniques either can be self-taught or learned from a therapist; in some cases,

Acute pain

severe, short-term pain.

Chronic or persistent pain

pain that is present for long periods of time, though not always at the same level of intensity.

Coping with Treatment and Side Effects

biofeedback machines, which monitor pulse and respiration, are used to teach people to concentrate on control of their breathing and heartbeat, which helps promote both concentration and relaxation. **Hypnosis,** a state of high concentration just on the edge of sleeping and wakefulness, is generally performed by someone else. A hypnotized person is highly receptive to suggestion and can be told by the hypnotist that the pain isn't there, effectively stopping, or at least reducing, the sensation of pain.

Hypnosis

a state of high concentration just on the edge of sleeping and wakefulness.

Other nonmedical techniques address some of the physical factors of pain. Heat and cold therapy, for example, uses the application of hot or cold packs to the areas where pain is felt to bring relief by redirecting the nerve impulses to bring messages other than pain sensations to the brain. Particularly where swelling or muscle tension occurs around the pain site, these therapies can also address some of the secondary causes of the pain by relieving those symptoms. Similarly, massage or shiatsu treatments can relieve muscle spasms and contractions and alleviate overall muscle tension. Other treatments include acupuncture, described in Question 55, and transcutaneous electric nerve stimulation (TENS), a technique that applies a mild electric current to the skin where the pain occurs. The current produces a pleasant sensation and relieves some types of pain. Physical therapy, particularly useful with regard to the arm and shoulder near the site of a mastectomy, helps return function and improve mobility; it can sometimes incorporate positioning techniques to relieve pressure on painful parts of the body and improve circulation.

Medical Pain Management

For mild pain, the first choice is usually medicines you can get from your medicine cabinet: acetaminophen (Tylenol) and any of a number of widely available **non-**

steroidal anti-inflammatory drugs (NSAIDs), which include aspirin, ibuprofen, naproxen sodium, and similar drugs available either over the counter or by prescription. Even though you may already be familiar with such drugs, you should consult your doctor before taking them, and be especially careful not to exceed the maximum daily dose on the label unless instructed otherwise by your doctor. The reason for this is simple: although they are safe for general non-prescription use when taken in accordance to the labels, even such common, generally safe pain medicines as acetaminophen can cause serious side effects if too much is taken for too long.

More severe pain usually requires treatment with stronger medicines available only by prescription—usually **opioids**, medicines derived from morphine and similar chemicals. These are available only by prescription because all opium derivatives are considered controlled substances and are strictly regulated by the FDA.

Some of the weaker opioids, including codeine and hydrocodone, are often mixed with acetaminophen or NSAIDs; stronger medications, such as morphine, hydromorphone, oxycodone, fentanyl, methadone, and levorphanol may have side effects that can limit the dose of the drug that can be given.

Other Treatment Methods

Localized pain that does not respond to drugs can sometimes be treated with a local anesthetic, usually combined with a steroid, which is injected into a nerve, nerve root, or spinal cord space to block pain. In other selected circumstances, the nerves may be surgically cut to block the pain. In instances when a nerve cannot be

Nonsteroidal anti-inflammatory drugs (NSAIDs)

a class of pain medications, often sold over the counter, that includes ibuprofen and similar common pain killers.

Opioids

medicines derived from morphine and similar chemicals.

Coping with Treatment and Side Effects

157

Table 7   Questions to Ask Your Doctor About Pain Control

✔ What can be done to relieve my pain?

✔ What can we do if the medicine doesn't work?

✔ What other options do I have for pain control?

✔ Will the pain medicines have side effects?

✔ What can be done to manage the side effects?

✔ Will the treatment limit my activities (i.e., working, driving, etc.)?

Source: National Comprehensive Cancer Network's Cancer Pain Treatment Guidelines for Patients. Reprinted by the permission of NCCN and the American Cancer Society. For additional information, contact the American Cancer Society and NCCN (see the appendix).

blocked, anesthesia can be achieved by injecting opioids into the spinal spaces using a pump to deliver a constant amount of drug.

The National Comprehensive Cancer Network, in association with the American Cancer Society, offers a booklet on pain relief for cancer patients, which can be obtained in printed or electronic form (see the appendix). In it, they suggest that patients talk to their doctors about pain relief using the questions listed in Table 7. These guidelines are also available from the American Cancer Society as part of a larger resource called *American Cancer Society's Guide to Pain Control: Powerful Methods to Overcome Cancer Pain* (see the appendix for ACS contact information).

58. What happens if the dose of pain medication I get isn't enough? Are pain drugs addictive?

Most cancer pain can be relieved if treated properly, but because of a number of myths and fears about pain management, many patients don't get the level of relief they need. Some patients, for example, fear that the side effects of the pain drugs will cause them additional discomfort. Opioid pain medications do have some side effects—most often, constipation, and occasionally nausea—but these side effects can be treated, usually with dietary adjustments such as increased fiber and fluids. Other patients feel that "suffering in silence" is somehow indicative of strength or stoic perseverance, thus they don't inform their doctor or nurses that they're experiencing pain. Still others feel that telling their doctor or nurse about pain is burdensome; they don't want to be a "bother" to the hospital staff. But there's no benefit to you or anyone else in your suffering—in fact, as noted in Question 57, negative experiences such as pain can suppress your immune system, so keeping quiet only decreases the weapons you have in fighting cancer. Pain also prevents you from doing whatever activities are still available, and it interferes with your enjoyment of your family and daily life. If you tell your doctors and nurses about your pain, you're not a whiner or a complainer—you're simply communicating to them the information they need to know to treat you effectively. They can't help you unless you tell them about the pain, and they do want to help—so don't be shy about telling them your concerns or problems with the medications they prescribe.

Most cancer pain can be relieved if treated properly, but many patients don't get the level of relief they need.

Fear of addiction on the part of the patient and, less frequently, the doctor or nurse, sometimes leads patients to take (or be given) a lower dose of opioid medications than is necessary to give the patient complete relief. Such fears are understandable: all of these medicines are derived from opium, which is highly addictive in itself. Yet fears of addiction are mostly exaggerated and represent a misunderstanding of the way a drug's addictive properties work. In part, this misunderstanding

Coping with Treatment and Side Effects

arises from confusion between addiction and an increase in medication tolerance—a situation in which a
certain level of medication no longer addresses the pain
felt by the patient. Tolerance is a common situation
with many kinds of medications, not simply pain drugs;
it means either that your body's response to the medication isn't as strong as it was at first, or that the factors
causing the pain are growing more severe, leading to a
higher level of pain than the current dose can affect. In
either case, you may need a higher dose or a different
medication—but you're not addicted to the medication
when this happens.

True addiction to the drug is a different situation altogether. A person can be addicted either physiologically
(a metabolic change occurs in the body) or psychologically (the person is obsessed with feeling the drug's effects in her body). Physiological addiction occurs when
the body's systems accept the presence of the medication as normal and necessary, so that the absence of it
causes symptoms such as cravings, tremors, sweats, and
pain—symptoms similar to those that true metabolic
imbalances might cause. Physiological addiction almost never occurs with cancer medications for two reasons: first, your need for pain medication usually is not
a continual situation (although, see the section on end-
of-life pain management), and second, the drugs are
working upon *abnormal* physiological episodes of pain
that the body cannot adjust to or accept as metabolical-
ly necessary. This doesn't mean that you'll instantly return to metabolic normality once your treatment for
cancer ends—you may have to reduce your pain medication gradually, as some of the factors stimulating
pain will continue for a time following treatment—but
it does mean that the drugs won't become a permanent

part of your body's physiological normality. Psychological addiction to cancer drugs also is uncommon, simply because the stimulus that causes you to take the drug—pain—is negative. People with psychological addictions generally want to experience the sensations that taking their drug brings—they're not looking for relief of pain, they're looking for the presence of a "high." Nevertheless, there are some people who need to be cautious about using pain medications, particularly those who are recovering from previous addictions to prescription or illegal drugs, so be sure to discuss any concerns in this regard with your doctor.

59. What can I do to deal with hair loss?

What any individual chooses to do about this problem is a matter of personal preference, but there are many options for coping with the emotional disturbance hair loss can cause. For example, you can prepare yourself for the possibility by getting a short haircut prior to beginning chemotherapy. Many women take this opportunity to shop for wigs that can take the place of natural hair for the duration of the chemotherapy, because it's important that you get fitted for your wig as soon as possible once you start losing your hair. Some insurance policies cover the purchase of wigs for cancer patients, so check to see what kind of insurance coverage you have. Also, your local American Cancer Society chapter may be able to provide a list of stores that sell wigs and other cosmetic aids or may have a collection of wigs given free of charge to cancer patients.

If wigs don't appeal to you, some cancer support groups offer fashion tips for using headscarves in lieu of wigs.

One that is of particular interest is the "Look Good, Feel Better" program jointly sponsored by the American Cancer Society and two beauty industry trade groups, the National Cosmetology Association and the Cosmetic, Toiletry, and Fragrance Association. This program offers seminars hosted by professional hairstylists and makeup artists to advise cancer patients on options for coping with hair loss and other side effects that treatment might have on their appearance. More information on this and similar programs is available in the appendix.

60. Do meditation and guided imaging really help prevent recurrences?

The reasons that cancer recurs are not well known, so it's difficult to determine what, if anything, can prevent recurrent cancer. Equally uncertain is the true extent of the power that the human mind has when it comes to healing or preventing disease. Yet as noted in previous discussions of these techniques, there is a definite benefit to using mind-body-spirit methods in marshaling the immune system against illness. It's doubtful that you can absolutely prevent recurrence should you practice meditation and guided imaging—there's no way of knowing, after all, whether or not you'd have had recurrence if you *didn't* meditate—but it may well increase your chances of avoiding another round of cancer. And even if you do practice these techniques and still have recurrent cancer, chances are good that you will be healthier in mind and spirit, and therefore more capable of fighting off the recurrence. So there's really nothing to lose and plenty to gain by practicing them—recurrence or no recurrence, you benefit by doing it.

You will be healthier in mind and spirit.

61. Where do I find treatment that will take a holistic approach to healing?

The National Institutes of Health's National Center for Complementary and Alternative Medicine (NCCAM) is just one resource for finding holistic health approaches. There's a clearinghouse of information on complementary and alternative medicine on their site (see the appendix). Telephone books usually list holistic health centers under "Holistic Practitioners," but be cautious about finding such centers that way—do some research about the places you find, talk to the physicians and patients there about how they practice, and make sure that any holistic practitioner you choose is able and willing to work with your medical team. Your own doctors may know such practitioners they've worked with before and can offer advice or referrals.

62. Do breast cancer support groups really help? Isn't the discussion depressing?

Discussion of cancer isn't nearly as depressing as facing it alone in isolation and fear. That's precisely why support groups really *do* help: they demystify the process of living with cancer, they help their members express the feelings that accompany the cancer diagnosis, and they give everyone in the group a chance to learn from the experiences of others who've walked in their shoes. One thing every cancer patient needs more than anything else is moral support: cancer treatment and recovery can be a long, difficult, emotionally draining process, and family and friends may be of help—but unless they've actually been through it themselves, they can't truly understand what it feels like to go through

Discussion of cancer isn't nearly as depressing as facing it alone in isolation and fear.

surgery, radiation, chemotherapy, or any combination of the three. Women in a cancer support group *know*; they've been through it and they truly empathize.

It's all very well for an outgoing person to wander into a room full of strangers and start talking about how it feels to have her breast removed, but what happens if you're an introvert? That's easy—you're not required to talk; you can learn just as much by listening. And if you find you don't care for the women in your group, then try another one—just don't give up on it. Once you start to feel familiar and comfortable with the women in your support group, you'll begin to gain a sense of sisterhood and encouragement, factors that might otherwise be in short supply at this point in your life. Yes, it may hurt at first to talk about everything you're going through, but the more you talk, the less it hurts, and the smaller the problem becomes.

You can usually find support groups through the hospital or cancer center you're using for your treatment, or by calling your local chapter of the American Cancer Society (see the appendix).

63. Can I put off surgery while I take an extended vacation?

You may have heard at some point of Dr. Jerri Nielsen, the woman doctor who volunteered to be part of the support staff for the Antarctic expedition run by the National Science Foundation, only to diagnose herself with an aggressive form of cancer when she was there. The drama of this situation was that Dr. Nielsen was isolated from treatment, and the possibility of getting to a place where she could get surgery and radiation therapy was limited by the harsh conditions of the Antarctic location. Ultimately, the risk to her life was great enough that a rescue team was sent to retrieve her despite the dangers of flying into the Antarctic during the winter. This effort was undertaken for one simple reason: where cancer is concerned, waiting is rarely a good idea; the time spent *not* getting treatment is time that the cancer has to grow and spread. If your cancer is advanced or aggressive, getting treatment as soon as possible is imperative, and any thoughts of a long vacation should be dismissed; if you've made a deposit on a cruise or airplane ticket, you probably can get the money back if you explain that it's a medical emergency (be prepared to have your doctor back you up with a letter, however). Even if you can't get a refund, however, you shouldn't go; your health is more important than any amount of money. What good is a Mediterranean cruise if going on it means you will return from it to face a more difficult treatment strategy and, possibly, death?

On the other hand, if your cancer is small and non-invasive, and you've made arrangements for a long trip that you've been anticipating for ages, it might be possible for you to take your trip, although a trip of more than a couple of weeks might have to be shortened. Discuss this question with your doctor to determine what he or she thinks about delaying surgery. If there are any concerns that the cancer could spread in the interim, you probably won't be able to go, but if the diagnosis indicates early-stage cancer—DCIS or LCIS—there's a possibility that your doctor will accept a delay.

Where cancer is concerned, waiting is rarely a good idea.

64. I can't afford the medicine for chemotherapy; can I use half the dose? Where can I find help with the expense if I don't have insurance?

The dose of medication prescribed by your doctor should never be altered; it was chosen for a reason and should be followed exactly. If you're having trouble paying for your medication, make sure your doctor knows of your situation; he may be able to substitute a generic drug or help you find a financial assistance program. If the problem is a limitation in your HMO or insurance benefits, check with your insurer to see if there is a "catastrophic illness" clause in your policy, which might be invoked to obtain additional funds for chemo drugs. Hospitals and clinics often have caseworkers or financial planners who can assist you in learning about and filing for additional benefits. There are also options if you don't have insurance coverage: government programs, disability benefits, services furnished by voluntary organizations, and others too numerous to mention. A good listing of the full variety of financial options can be obtained through the American Cancer Society, which offers the following advice to cancer patients with regard to dealing with insurance issues:

- Become familiar with your individual insurance plan and its provisions. If you think you might need additional insurance, ask your insurance carrier whether it is available.
- Submit claims for all medical expenses even when you are uncertain about your coverage.
- Keep accurate and complete records of claims submitted, pending, and paid.

- Keep copies of all paperwork related to your claims, such as letters of medical necessity, bills, receipts, requests for sick leave, and correspondence with insurance companies.
- Get a caseworker, a hospital financial counselor, or a social worker to help you if your finances are limited. Often, companies or hospitals can work with you to make acceptable payment arrangements if you make them aware of your situation.
- Submit your bills as you receive them. If you become overwhelmed with bills, get help. Contact local support organizations, such as your American Cancer Society or your state's government agencies, for additional assistance.
- Do not allow your medical insurance to expire. Pay premiums in full and on time. It is often difficult to get new insurance.

(Source: American Cancer Society's Web site, www. cancer.org. Reprinted with the permission of the American Cancer Society, Inc.)

This advice is worth following even if you don't have insurance. The better your recordkeeping, the more likely it will be that you can obtain financial assistance from either the government or private agencies.

Government Assistance

There are numerous government programs to assist with medical costs. If your income is below a set level, you may be eligible for Medicaid. Your state Medicaid office can tell you whether you're eligible, but if you aren't, it should be able to supplement at least part of the expense of your medications. States also usually have their own medical assistance programs for individuals below a certain income level, and many of these specifically address prescription drug costs; you can learn about these from a hospital social worker or case manager. There are also individual hospitals and clinics that receive funding from the federal government under the Hill-Burton Program, which helps these facilities to provide free or low-cost services. Ask your caseworker if your facility falls within these guidelines and can offer assistance. If you served in the armed forces, you may be eligible for veteran's benefits. The nature of these benefits changes frequently, so contact the Department of Veterans Affairs for information on what assistance you can get from them.

If you're not able to work, find out whether you qualify for disability, either through a long-term disability insurance policy (which some companies offer to their employees as a benefit) or through Social Security. The Social Security Administration should be able to tell you whether you qualify—and if they turn you down the first time, reapply, because it's not unusual for cases to be approved after an appeal. Benefits will start 6 months after the start of qualifying disability, so be sure you carefully document when you ceased being able to work with corroborating details from your doctor. You may also be able to get Supplemental Security Income (SSI) if your income was very low prior to your becoming disabled, you're over 65, or you're blind. SSI varies from state to state, but even a small subsidy to your monthly income could provide substantial help in paying for medications.

Private Assistance

Many private organizations offer financial assistance and services for cancer patients and their families. One source of assistance might surprise you: the drug companies that manufacture these expensive medications sometimes provide assistance to those patients who can't pay for their prescriptions. Check with your doctor or individual drug companies to find out whether they have any programs for which you may be eligible. Private charitable foundations, civic or religious bodies, and similar organizations provide financial assistance and services; the American Cancer Society, listed in the appendix, is just one. Many others—the United Way, the Salvation Army, and religious social services of particular denominations—can be found in the phone book under "Social Services." If you're a member of a union, contact your local chapter and ask whether they have any resources you can tap.

Whatever options you choose, remember that curing your cancer is the most important thing. Don't deprive yourself of your medication because of limited resources; instead, look for additional resources to help pay for the pills. You may be surprised at how much is out there for someone who takes the time to look for it.

65. Can I use something for nausea from the chemotherapy? Does marijuana help me find relief?

The medical marijuana controversy is ongoing, but it boils down to one issue: should this illegal drug be made available to cancer patients for relief of pain and nausea? Advocates of legalization for medical purposes claim that marijuana, or "pot," is superior to traditional medicines in relieving these symptoms. Most studies of the active ingredient in marijuana, a chemical called THC, show that when administered in pure form, it gives no greater relief than approved medications. Smoking pot also introduces all the complications of smoking anything—you're inhaling smoke and particulate matter into the lungs, which is never good for you and can cause serious health complications in light of your ongoing battle against cancer. Take into account as well that regardless of why you're using it, possession of marijuana is still a crime for which you can go to jail, and the risks of using it far outweigh the questionable benefits.

Nausea from chemotherapy is treatable using nutrition and legal medications (see Question 49). Talk to your doctor and nutritionist for help in controlling nausea.

66. I got my diagnosis through Medicaid. Will Medicaid also cover my treatment?

The Breast and Cervical Cancer Prevention and Treatment Act passed by Congress in 2000 gives the states options for follow-up treatment services through Medicaid. At least 20 states have signed on to this program, with more expected to follow. For a woman to be eligible for Medicaid under this option, she must have been screened for and found to have breast or cervical cancer, including precancerous conditions, through the National Breast and Cervical Cancer Early Detection Program (NBCCEDP); be under age 65; and be uninsured and otherwise not eligible for Medicaid. Check with your state's health department to find out whether your state participates if you qualify.

67. When all else fails, how do I prepare myself and my family for my death?

Too few people think ahead to what happens should cancer get the better of them. Even knowing that breast cancer is one of the top killers of women over 40, most people prefer to concentrate instead on curing the cancer—an understandable attitude that is to be encouraged. As time passes and the cancer advances, however, there comes a point when cancer patients should start thinking about what they want to have happen should they lose the battle. As difficult as it might be to contemplate your own death, doing so before the end is imminent can ease matters for you and your family when you do finally reach that point—if you ever do. Everyone hopes that they'll never need such arrangements any time soon, but if you work out ahead of time (while you're still feeling relatively good) the details of wills, power of attorney designation, DNR (do not resuscitate) orders, funeral arrangements, and similar practical matters, it is easier to focus on your health knowing that these structures are in place should they become necessary. There are several steps you can take to accomplish this.

Work toward acceptance. Even after a long, difficult illness, it's very hard to accept that you're going to die within the next few months or weeks. Preparing yourself for death is perhaps the greatest emotional and spiritual undertaking of your life, so get assistance from a minister, social worker, or psychologist. If you don't have a minister or counselor with whom you're comfortable, most cancer centers or oncology wards have a chaplain or counselor in residence. Take advantage of their services, or ask for a referral. Involve your family in some of these sessions, but reserve as many as you need for yourself—if you can gain a sense of peace for yourself, it will help your family to cope with your death too. Ironically, achieving this sort of peace and acceptance can help you to live longer than predicted. It's not unknown for people thought to have only a few

Ironically, achieving this sort of peace and acceptance can help you to live longer than predicted.

months remaining to live many months, even years, after making their "final" arrangements for death.

Many people find this time hard to think about and talk about, and it's likely that you'll have to raise the issue with your family, friends, and health care team. Your loved ones may resist the discussion, but be persistent—or get help from a counselor or minister who can guide them through this painful conversation. It's important to talk about what you want to happen in the final phases of your illness. Discuss the organization of personal documents and where you keep them so that your family and friends know where they are and what your wishes and desires are. Lawyers, clergy, and counselors may also help you and your family in planning for end-of-life issues.

Decide on the best place for your care. People coping with advanced cancer have choices for the location of their care: in the home, in an outpatient setting or the doctor's office, in the hospital, or through a hospice. Although a person can live with recurrent or metastatic disease for a long time, people with advanced disease will reach a point where it becomes clear that they are dying. It may be best to discuss these choices prior to this point, if you can. Hospice care focuses on improving the quality of life for the remainder of your life and can make the dying process as comfortable and pain free as possible. Hospice care can be given in the home, the hospital, or in a separate hospice. These are all personal choices based on your needs and available resources. Your health care team can discuss these options with you and help you get the care you need.

Make your wishes known. If cancer treatment becomes unbearable, you have the right to request that your doctors stop treatment. You even have the ability to describe in writing what kinds of treatment you will and will not accept from them in case you should lose the ability to communicate your wishes directly. Legal documents called **advance directives**, including living wills, durable power of attorney, DNR orders, and health care proxies, allow people to express their decisions regarding what is acceptable to them during their last weeks or months in case they become unable to communicate effectively. These are described in Question 68.

Advance directives

legal documents that allow people to express their decisions regarding what they do and don't want to have done during their last weeks or months in case they become unable to communicate effectively.

68. Are there legal steps I can take to make my wishes known in case I'm not able to speak for myself near the end?

You have the right to decide what treatment you will and will not accept near the end of your life. You also have the right to designate an individual to speak for you—usually a member of your family, but it can be a friend or an attorney. You don't need an official document or form—you don't even need to have this document written by an attorney. All you really need to do is sign a letter in the presence of two or more witnesses (who should also sign and date the document), although if you have the letter notarized it will carry more weight with a hospital board.

Advance directives dictating how you want your treatment to proceed include living wills, DNR orders, durable power of attorney, and health care proxies. A **living will** simply outlines what care you want in the event that you become unable to communicate due to coma or heavy sedation. You're not locked into anything you write down—the document is simply a legally valid guide for families and physicians to know a patient's thinking about how she should be cared for, and

Living will

a document that outlines what care you want in the event that you become unable to communicate due to coma or heavy sedation.

should you change your mind about any of it, you can change the directives or even verbally countermand them to the physician treating you. Alternatively, you can limit the instructions to a *do not resuscitate order* (DNR) if you want, telling the medical staff at the hospital that they should not act to revive you should your heart or brain activity stop.

Even if you don't write it down, if you have certain ideas as to what kind of treatment you do and don't want, all you need to do is tell members of your family, particularly those acting as your principal caregivers. If they know your wishes, they can intervene on your behalf even without a written statement—though they may have to convince a judge that this is truly your wish, should the hospital balk at their requests to withhold treatment. In such cases, your family will be bolstered if you prepare, in advance, a **durable power of attorney** (which allows a specific family member to legally make all your decisions, personal and financial, for you in case you become incapacitated) or a **health care proxy**, which limits the designated person's decision-making power to only those decisions regarding your medical treatment.

Durable power of attorney

allows a specific family member to legally make all your decisions, personal and financial, for you in case you become incapacitated.

Health care proxy

permits a designated person to make decisions regarding your medical treatment when you are unable to do so.

If you don't have a will, you should write one as soon as possible, particularly if you have children. Should you fail to do this, most states' laws arrange for your assets to go directly to your spouse and children in specific proportions, but processing your estate will take considerably more time, potentially causing problems for your family if bank accounts, property, or savings were solely in your name. And where circumstances might have created other mitigating factors—prior marriages with or without children, common-law marriages or other nontraditional relationships—having a will clarifies your wishes and is a tremendous kindness to your loved ones. Some people also make advance arrangements for their funerals, which can be particularly helpful to your family, as they won't have to work out these details in the midst of their grief over your death. Doing so might be difficult—there is no more stark confrontation with your impending mortality than arranging your own funeral—but it can also help bring a measure of acceptance and peace knowing you have taken care of this important detail ahead of time.

PART SIX

Changes Cancer Brings

How do I get my life back to normal?

Is it normal not to have mood swings when diagnosed, or will there be a delay in that response?

How does cancer affect sexuality, intimacy, and fertility?

More ...

YOUR EMOTIONS

69. How do I get my life back to normal?

Cancer diagnosis, treatment, and even recovery are all experiences that will change your life permanently. You can pretend the change didn't happen, and you can go back to the same activities you were doing before your diagnosis, but it doesn't change a thing—and your body knows it, even if your mind and heart don't want to admit it. You may go through some major emotional changes (see Questions 70, 72, and 73 for more on this subject) but sooner or later, you will understand that there's no going back to your old normality. However, that doesn't necessarily have to be a *bad* thing. Many cancer survivors realize that treatment has given them a "new lease on life" both physically and emotionally. It's shown them things they were missing in their lives, ways to prioritize that make them happier, even given them habits that improve the structure of their day-to-day relationships with people, work, community, and most of all, themselves. If a wholesale overhaul of your existence sounds like a big project, the good news is, there are people and organizations out there to help you restructure your life: you don't have to do it alone.

Many cancer survivors realize that treatment has given them a "new lease on life" both physically and emotionally.

Think carefully about how you ran your life prior to your diagnosis. Were you truly happy? Did you take care of yourself, not just physically but also emotionally and spiritually? Were you close with your partner, your family, your friends? Were there things you always meant to do in your life—traveling, concerts, visits to relatives, and so on—that you put off because you simply didn't get around to it?

Cancer forces patients to reprioritize their lives, because the demands of treatment abruptly come first.

Cancer forces patients to reprioritize their lives.

Suddenly, you find yourself obliged to let things slide that used to be your top concern—you have to really think about what in your life is crucial and what isn't. Maybe you find this enforced assessment frustrating, but it can also be an opportunity to change aspects of your life that you weren't satisfied with before your diagnosis. When treatment ends and you're "clean," it's a good time to think about what you'd *really* like to put first. Maybe you want to spend more time with your partner or children—it could mean altering your job circumstances, changing to part-time work, or getting a home computer so you can telecommute a few days a week. Perhaps it's time to take a few weeks of vacation time for that long-overdue trip to Hawaii. Maybe it means something as simple as signing up for a yoga class to learn new relaxation techniques or going to church more often to reconnect with your spiritual upbringing. Whatever it could mean for you, "getting *back* to normal" involves developing a *forward*-looking attitude. Cancer has brought changes to your life; it's up to you to make them positive changes to create a new, better "normal."

70. Is it normal not to have mood swings when diagnosed, or will there be a delay in that response?

Everyone's response to the diagnosis is different, so there's really no such thing as a *normal* response. Yes, many patients do experience mood swings when they hear they have cancer, but others don't; it really depends on your ability to absorb and cope with bad news. Some people respond with denial—they try to ignore the changes, but it gets awfully hard to do that when you're in the midst of chemotherapy-induced nausea. Others get angry: what did I do to deserve this? The answer is obvious, when you think about it: you did nothing wrong, you *don't* deserve it, but it's not a question of what you do or don't deserve—it's something that just happened, and getting mad about it doesn't change a thing. You might feel many emotions, some right away, some a little bit later. At first, you might not feel anything; a feeling of numbness or emotional paralysis isn't uncommon, but if it persists beyond a short time—a week or two—you may want to talk to a social worker, therapist, or minister, because one thing you can't afford to do is let your life just halt. You're ill, you need treatment, and most of all, you need to proceed with your life if you want to beat this disease.

The most important thing regarding your emotional response is that you deal with it appropriately. Don't ignore your emotions—bottling them up simply makes matters worse, and you could find yourself getting angry or upset in unexpected and unhealthy ways. You don't want to take your anger out on your children or your spouse—that helps no one and hurts everyone, including you. Whatever feelings you have, get them out somehow, whether it be through writing in a journal or talking—to your spouse, a friend, a relative, a minister, or a counselor. Support groups are invaluable in this respect because everyone there has been through, or is going through, what you're experiencing right now, so they'll not only understand perfectly what it's like, they may have excellent advice on how to cope. See Question 62 for more on support groups.

*Don't ignore
your emotions.*

71. *What role do past pain, anger, stress, and fear play in this disease?*

The impact of negative emotions on the body is an intriguing topic. Do negative emotions make a person sick? In a way, they do—indirectly. Cancer, as we know, is uncontrolled cellular division caused by a mutation. The mutation has nothing to do with emotions—it's something that a person is born with or that happened by accident in her cells. Where the emotions come into the picture is in two body systems, responsive to emotions, that can affect the cancer's spread: the endocrine (hormonal) system and the immune system.

Do negative emotions make a person sick?

Everyone's heard of the wild mood swings sometimes caused by the fluctuations in hormones caused by pregnancy—they even happen in some women in the context of the menstrual cycle. It works similarly in reverse, though not quite to the same extent: emotions, both positive and negative, affect the hormones. For instance, severe stress or depression can suppress estrogen and/or progesterone levels to the point at which a woman's menstrual periods stop altogether. Such emotions also raise levels of certain stress-related hormones, which in turn suppress the immune system. Positive emotions, on the other hand, tend to contribute to more consistent hormone levels and boost the immune system. In the presence of positive emotions, the body's systems tend to work more smoothly and efficiently.

Scientific studies of whether depressed or anxious women get breast cancer more often than women who have neutral or positive emotional histories have had mixed results: while some have shown a link between a breast cancer diagnosis and a history of depression, others have found no such correlation. Does this mean that past feelings of depression or anger "caused" your cancer? No, and it's important that this distinction is understood because many women feel guilty about having "done something" to have contributed to their current situation. If you are mired in negative emotions, it seems logical that you'd be more susceptible to cancer simply because your immune system is suppressed, but you're just as likely—or more likely—to have gotten a bad cold, the flu, or any other illness in such a situation. The fact that cancer, and not a more easily treated illness, was the disease that took advantage of your lowered defenses is nothing more than bad luck.

If you look back on your life prediagnosis and see a great deal of negativity, emotions that you now regret and fear that could have contributed to your illness, don't dwell on it—you can't change what's in the past. What you *can* do is change the present and the future: find ways to encourage a more positive outlook in yourself. This can be as simple as taking time to do things you enjoy, or it can involve visiting a therapist or a minister to talk about your negative attitude and find ways to change. The benefits of taking such steps include not only the potential to boost the immune system, but also an improved quality to your life, even in the face of the difficulties of cancer treatment. Question 60 gives more information on mind-over-body techniques that can help to improve immune response and quality of life.

You can't change what's in the past.

72. Since my diagnosis of cancer, I'm not able to concentrate. Why is this happening? Is there anything I can do about it?

In a word: *stress*. Poor concentration is a classic symptom of high levels of stress in anyone, cancer patient or not. It's perfectly understandable too—you've just received the shock of a lifetime and your world is turned upside down. Poor ability to concentrate is normal under these circumstances.

There are any number of methods to address this problem. A classic way to relieve stress is exercise. It doesn't have to mean signing up for aerobics classes at the local gym—regular walks in the park will do, as the main point is to get your body moving, even if only a little bit. Exercise may be difficult for you, however, if you're suffering from severe fatigue or nausea associated with treatment; a less physically strenuous method is to make use of mental relaxation techniques, such as **meditation** and **guided imagery** (described in brief in Question 55). Many cancer centers offer classes or group sessions to teach relaxation and meditation techniques; if yours does not, ask your doctor or nurse for a referral to one that does, or check with the National Center for Complementary and Alternative Medicine (NCCAM) at the National Institutes of Health to find links to locations offering such services. You don't necessarily have to attend a class, however; meditation can be done simply by concentrating your mind on an inanimate object—a rock, for instance—and focusing on it to the exclusion of all else, clearing the mind of worries, fears, and the millions of inane thoughts that cross our minds each minute. Alternatively, you can meditate on spiritual or religious teachings, many of which are offered in books that provide a topic for each day. This may take a little bit of practice—don't be discouraged if you can't master it the first few days you try it. Another possibility is to use relaxation techniques that combine physical activity with meditation, such as yoga, tai chi, or qi gong; classes in these techniques are widely available and can often be found through your

Mediation

a mental technique that clears the mind and relaxes the body through concentration.

Guided imagery

a mind–body technique in which the patient visualizes and meditates upon images that encourage a positive immune response.

local YMCA or church, or simply by looking through the yellow pages.

Talk to your doctor about the difficulties you're having, too—there are some chemotherapy regimens that contribute to mental confusion, and it may be that this is as much a pharmacological problem as an emotional one. Although it might not mean changing the regimen, there could be ways of reducing the problem—altering the timing of your medication, for instance, so you take it later in the day or at night, leaving you better able to concentrate during your normal daily activities. You could also be suffering from depression, which can be treated.

73. How does one stop thinking about a cancer diagnosis? Why does the cancer diagnosis appear to be more frightening at night?

You can't stop thinking about your cancer diagnosis altogether—ignoring it won't make it go away, and you still have to go through treatment—but it doesn't have to rule your life. Yet at night, when you've settled into bed and there are no tasks at hand to distract you, you may find yourself turning the diagnosis over and over in your head, wondering how this could happen to you. What did you do that might have caused this? What are you going to do now? How will the treatment change your life? Is it going to be painful? What if it can't be cured? What if you lose your job?

It doesn't have to rule your life.

Worrying about the many effects of a cancer diagnosis is perfectly natural, but it can be exhausting. More to the point, it diverts valuable energy from the process of regaining your health. One method that could help is to make a commitment to yourself that you'll limit your "worry time" to a specific time or place each day; perhaps a half hour just before lunchtime, but try to avoid the evening hours prior to bedtime. Then get it all out—worry away—and try to either devise constructive solutions to your concerns or figure out where to get such solutions. Make lists of questions and fears and present them to your medical team, a therapist, a minister—whoever you think is most appropriate to help you answer them. And when your worry time is done for that day, it's done—no more allowed until tomorrow. If you find yourself unable to enforce this restriction, get help from a therapist or a minister trained in dealing with the emotional impact of cancer. Again, meditation and relaxation techniques as described in Questions 55 and 72 may help.

74. Should I take leave from a highly stressful job while I'm going through treatment?

There are advantages and disadvantages to considering taking a leave of absence from your work. Talk to your doctor frankly about what effects your diagnosis and treatment may have upon your ability to work, and then discuss with your employer how to handle changes that might occur in your ability to function. If continuing to work while you're undergoing treatment is exhausting or you find that your ability to do a good job is compromised by fatigue or other symptoms, you may be better off leaving the job for a few months to concentrate on your health. Most full-time workers covered by group health benefits are entitled to 12 weeks of unpaid leave (with continuing health benefits) by the Family and Medical Leave Act (FMLA). Your job is protected for the duration of your leave, so you don't need to fear losing it. As a cancer patient, you are also entitled to protections provided by the Americans with Disabilities Act (ADA), which is administered by the Equal Employment Opportunity Commission (EEOC). Be sure to familiarize yourself with both laws prior to approaching your employer.

If your treatment isn't debilitating but you have enough difficulties that you can't work full time, you may want to try to find an alternative to leaving altogether. Depending on your circumstances, you may be able to get a reduction in workload, arrange to telecommute certain days of the week, or change, temporarily, to part-time status. Discuss these options with your employer or human resources director; most will be sympathetic and flexible.

If you're not eligible for the FMLA, there are other ways you can arrange a leave of absence. Again, talk to your employer about ways to work around the effects of treatment, bearing in mind that you are covered by the ADA even if the FMLA doesn't apply, which means you can't be fired just for being sick. If you and your employer can't arrange a compromise on a workload adjustment, there are government resources available to provide financial assistance while you're undergoing treatment. Check with the Social Security Administration—sometimes your benefits can be released before the age of eligibility if you're facing illness-related financial strains. Many utility companies also have programs to offset the costs of heat, electricity, and other expenses during episodes of serious illness, so contact your local utilities as well.

75. How do I cope with the fear of recurrence?

There are several ways you can address your fear. One is by talking to other people who have been where you are—join a support group or take part in online chat rooms. Just expressing your feelings about this concern can alleviate some of the anxiety. You can also speak to a therapist or minister about these fears to get some emotional or spiritual support in handling them. See Question 62 for more on support groups.

Another way is by taking steps to improve your overall health: once you've recovered from the effects of your treatment, work towards better health habits and a stronger body. Many of the suggestions in Question 72 can be utilized against fear in addition to stress. Improve your daily nutrition and exercise habits, quit smoking (if you smoke), lower your alcohol intake, and practice relaxation techniques such as meditation.

YOUR BODY

76. My body seems different now that I have cancer—I don't feel as attractive. What can I do to change this?

Our culture has traditionally stressed breasts as a fundamental part of feminine beauty and sexuality, so losing one or both breasts to cancer can be traumatic. It's not unusual for women, even women who were confident about their attractiveness prior to their mastectomy, to feel insecure about their sexuality after losing a breast.

There are several ways to approach this problem. Breast reconstruction (see Question 39) restores the shape of the breast, but cannot restore normal breast sensation. With time, the skin on the reconstructed breast becomes more sensitive, but it will never be the same as before the mastectomy. Breast reconstruction often makes women more comfortable with their bodies, however, and helps them feel more attractive. If you opted against reconstructing your breast initially, but find that you've changed your mind, talk to your doctor—reconstruction is still a viable option.

Alternatively, you can approach the feelings of insecurity from the inside, through counseling. A therapist can help you to adjust and accept the changes that have occurred in your body, so that the loss of the breast doesn't affect your image of yourself as beautiful. Indeed, there are some women who adopt the stance that society's view of breasts as essential to feminine beauty is something they can reject by accepting their body as it is, with or without breasts.

These options work well when dealing with one's confidence strictly in the sense of public personal appearance. But what do you do when you have to show your body to a husband or partner? Particularly on the first occasion that your husband or lover sees you after the surgery, it can be extremely uncomfortable. Moreover, the breasts and nipples are sources of sexual pleasure for many women. Touching the breasts is a common part of sexual intimacy in our culture. After a mastectomy, the whole breast is gone—it's not something you can hide or disguise. How do you deal with that?

Part 7 offers more specific advice on how to deal with sexuality after a mastectomy, but it's important to note here that the only way to mitigate discomfort or embarrassment is to make sure both you and your partner are prepared for what you're going to see and experience on the first viewing of your changed body. Talk about it beforehand as much as you need to—with a relationship or marriage counselor if you find that simple one-on-one discussion is too awkward at first—and continue to be open with your partner as you begin to reacquaint yourselves with the changes to your body. The first time you're intimate with your partner might bring on many difficult emotions or revive feelings you thought were done with—anger, fear, "why me?"—so be prepared for what might be a difficult encounter, but remember that with time and compassion from each of you to one another, the discomfort will eventually pass.

77. Should I tell someone taking my blood pressure that I have had a mastectomy on that side?

Absolutely, you should, particularly if the mastectomy was performed within the past few years. Some clinicians think that use of a blood pressure cuff on the side you've had your mastectomy can trigger lymphedema, although this has not been proven. This effect is not limited to the period immediately after your surgery, but can last as long as several years. You should do what you can to avoid this complication, and that includes protecting your arm from injury and pressure—even the minor pressure of a blood pressure cuff. Question 41 has a complete description of what lymphedema is and how to prevent it.

78. Does liposuction work to make my breasts the same size?

No. Liposuction is a technique that removes fat from an area under the skin, and your healthy breast is composed of far more than just fat—there are muscles and breast tissue and structures among the fat cells in the breast. Moreover, liposuction carries with it the possibility of infection, which your overstressed immune system may not be able to handle very well. If your breasts are greatly irregular in size following surgery, you should consult with a plastic surgeon about **breast-reduction surgery**, which removes not only fat, but breast tissue as well, to make the other breast match the breast that has been surgically altered. But be careful: although reconstructive surgery is usually covered by insurance, breast-reduction surgery is considered a cosmetic procedure and probably won't be.

Breast-reduction surgery

removes not only fat, but breast tissue as well, to make the contralateral breast match the breast that has been surgically altered.

79. Does positive thinking have any power in the healing process? How do I motivate myself?

In Question 71, we discussed how negative thinking can depress the immune system, leaving the body more vulnerable to diseases, including cancer. The flip side of this is the question of whether women with more cheerful attitudes are less likely to get cancer. They're not, but they have a better prognosis when they do get it. Positive thinking does affect the healing process, and it can be an important component in battling cancer. The cliché that "laughter is the best medicine" exists precisely because people who are happy, who enjoy life, who have fun, tend to be healthier than those who don't. Not only do happy people tend to take better care of themselves and eat better, they also recover more quickly from illness. The reason for this is simple: happy people get an immune boost simply by being happy. The rule of thumb, as determined by immune researchers, is that a positive event can boost the immune system for up to three days, whereas a negative one can suppress it for a day. But whether an event is

Positive thinking does affect the healing process.

positive or negative depends largely on a person's perspective: to some very cheerful people, just walking out the door on a beautiful fall day can be an extremely positive experience, whereas a depressed or angry person might not even see the sunlight, thus missing out on the immune boost experienced by the happy person.

Motivating oneself to think positively can be tricky to one who may not be accustomed to it, but the key is to make it habitual. Choose a specific time each day to do something nice for yourself. Listen to music, look at pictures, pet your dog, rent a movie, or even just sit down in a quiet place and meditate on things that make you happy—playing with your children, stroking your pets, traveling to Paris, eating ice cream, shopping for shoes. It doesn't matter what you use, so long as doing or thinking about it makes you feel good. Above all, don't neglect this time—take it as seriously as you would the need to take your chemo pills, because the goal is the same.

There are amazing stories of what people can accomplish through mind-over-matter techniques, simply by cultivating a positive attitude. Cancer patients given a prognosis of death within months have been known to defy these predictions by years, even decades. Most of them accomplished this feat through positive thinking—so give yourself a pep talk: "I'm going to beat this thing, and I'm going to enjoy doing it!" Picture yourself beating it, not just in terms of having a victory, but in *literal* terms, whacking it with a stick. Go a step further—get a pillow or stuffed animal, call it "cancer," and whack it with a stick as hard as you can. Sounds silly? Certainly it does, but similar techniques have worked for many cancer patients. It can help you release tension, frustration, and anger associated with your diagnosis and treatment—you might even find it fun!—and if the worst thing that happens is that you feel ridiculous, you're no worse off than you were.

YOUR FAMILY

80. Why is it so difficult to tell friends and loved ones about my cancer diagnosis?

Cancer is difficult enough to accept when you hear the diagnosis from your doctor. Yet somehow, telling the people you care about is even more difficult. There are a number of reasons for this: first, telling people about the diagnosis makes it seem that much more "real" to you at a time when you might still be wishing that it wasn't real. Saying repeatedly, "I have breast cancer" to various family and friends effectively drills this fact into your mind—and who wouldn't prefer to pretend that this wasn't the case?

Second, telling your friends and loved ones is painful because you have to see their reactions, which might mirror your own: shock, fear, and grief. Many newly diagnosed patients feel guilt at causing these emotions in people they love, which makes them all the more reluctant to tell their family and friends. There's also a certain level of fear that your loved ones, knowing you have cancer, may distance themselves from you—it hasn't been that long since cancer was instinctively identified as automatically terminal. You may also have practical concerns about job security—will you get fired or demoted if your boss believes your illness or treatment interferes with your productivity?

It might seem that hiding the truth is your best strategy, but be practical: it's physically impossible to keep the truth from those closest to you. You're going to have surgery, probably also a round of radiation or chemotherapy, and the effects of these treatments will be highly visible, particularly if your cancer is advanced. Sooner or later, they'll know something's wrong—and if any of them have ever had a friend or relative with cancer (you'd be amazed at how many have seen it before), they'll quickly figure out what's up. Hiding the truth will accomplish nothing positive and will do much damage to your relationships with your loved ones. Your friends and family may feel deceived and hurt, and you'll lose the good will of the people you most need to support you during your treatment.

For those closest to you—your spouse or partner, your parents, your siblings, your best friend—it's probably best to tell them yourself. For others who may be more distant, you may be able to enlist the assistance of a friend or relative to pass the news along. With respect to your employer, you should definitely be honest about your illness because treatment may require taking a leave of absence; if the employment situation is difficult enough that you're concerned about losing the job, it might be time to consider your financial position and decide whether leaving the job altogether is the right strategy (see Question 74).

The National Cancer Institute's CancerNet service summarizes the reasons for being open with your loved ones admirably:

- Cancer can be unutterably lonely. No one should try to bear it alone.
- Most people find it easier for all if everybody can share their feelings instead of hiding them. This frees people to offer each other support.

- Families say patients who try to keep the diagnosis secret rob loved ones of the chance to express their love and to offer help and support.
- Family members and intimate friends also bear great emotional burdens and should be able to share them openly with each other and the patient.
- Even children should be told. They sense when something is amiss, and they may imagine a situation worse than it really is (see Question 84.)
- The patient might want to tell the children directly, or it may be easier to have a close friend or loving relative do so.
- The children's ages and emotional maturity should be a guide in deciding how much to tell. The goal is to let children express their feelings and ask questions about the cancer.
- By sharing the diagnosis, patient, family, and friends build foundations of mutual understanding and trust.

The bottom line is this: the people closest to you are the ones who are going to drive you to your doctor's appointments when you're feeling weak and nauseous; the ones who will make your meals, pick up your medications from the pharmacy, and take your children to school when you're too fatigued to do it; and they're the ones you'll talk to when you need encouragement and companionship. Don't make their job any more difficult by not telling them what they need to know from the outset.

81. What support system is available for my family?

Cancer isn't something that just affects you—it affects all the people in your life, including your spouse, your children, your extended family, and your friends. They may not have a good understanding of what cancer

Cancer affects all the people in your life.

means, and like you, they have many different reactions—feelings of fear, anger, denial. They may find it hard to be supportive of you because they're struggling with their own emotions. Furthermore, they may find it difficult to give you the time and energy you're going to need. If your spouse works 14-hour days, for instance, he may not have the energy to drive you to your chemotherapy sessions. The key is to find ways to help your family to work with this difficult situation. That could mean using one of many strategies:

- **Don't refuse offers of assistance:** Members of your extended family, friends, or coworkers may offer their assistance; "If there's anything I can do to help, just let me know," is a common response when a friend is in need. It might be second nature to simply reply, "Thank you, but it's under control," yet this is your opportunity to obtain some relief for your family that you may not yet realize they're going to need. Break the habit of automatically refusing; make sure that anyone who makes this offer understands that you may need to take them up on it. Even people you don't know very well may be willing to do things like help with yard work, take your car for an oil change or fill-up, and similar small but necessary tasks.

- **Find ways to adjust the household routine so it doesn't overburden your family:** You may not be able to do as much around the house if your treatment causes you to become tired and nauseous, but family members picking up the slack may become tired and overstressed. Think about the tasks that must get done and find ways to minimize them. For instance, if you used to do all the grocery shopping, you might get a shopping service to do this instead of asking your partner to take on the additional task. House cleaning, laundry, and similar tasks can all be done by commercial services—perhaps not all the time, but on occasion.

- **Find assistance with child care:** You don't have to hire a nanny just because you're sick—it could be as simple as taking advantage of school-based before- or after-school programs, or asking a relative or friend to pick the children up after school a few days a week. Some local YMCAs will pick up children at school and take them to a central facility where the kids can do homework and participate in activities for several hours. You may find that having the extra time helps you to balance the demands of your family and your illness better, and the costs associated with this program may be tax deductible.

- **Consider a leave of absence from work—for either you or your spouse:** Under the Family and Medical Leave Act, either you or your spouse may be able to take a 12-week unpaid leave of absence from your job, depending on whether your work situation qualifies. To determine whether one or both of you are eligible, check the Department of Labor Web site's FMLA page (http://*www.dol.gov/elaws/fmla.html*).

- **Take advantage of support programs for cancer patients:** The American Cancer Society has a number of programs aimed at cancer patients in general and breast cancer patients specifically. The Road to Recovery program, for instance, offers rides to treatment sessions, while the I Can Cope service provides a series of seminars on how you and your family can adjust to life with cancer. Other similar programs are widely available; ask your doctor for referral, or contact your local ACS chapter for more information.

82. Is there a way for me to talk to my children about cancer without frightening them?

There are a few rules of thumb when talking to your children about cancer. First, as tempting as it might be to say nothing about your illness so you won't upset them, *don't exclude them*. This recommendation extends to children of any age, whether they be preschoolers or adults with families of their own: if you leave them out of the loop, they will not only feel hurt or deeply resentful, but you will also lose out on the assistance, support, and love they have to offer you. During the treatment stage, when side effects can become debilitating, you will need as much support and assistance as you can get from those around you, including your children, grown or not. Even in cases where you and your children are estranged, it's important that you give them the information so they can decide whether to put aside their differences with you and offer help. They may not, and telling them could change nothing—but *not* telling them will only hurt matters. Using a relative, a member of the clergy, or a mutual friend as a go-between could be one option if there is a very serious rift between you and your children. But if you're not on speaking terms, your best bet might be to have your doctor write a letter explaining your condition; this could prevent any suspicions that you might be manipulating them or trying to make them feel guilty, as well as transmitting the bare facts of your condition without any emotional baggage attached.

With children still young enough to live at home, hiding the truth really is not an option, no matter how hard you might try. They will know that something's wrong with

Mom—it's unavoidable—and not knowing *what* is wrong will be far more damaging to them than knowing. Though most of your energy will be focused on your treatment, as their parent you have the responsibility to allay as much of their anxiety as possible. For pre-teen children, a second rule of thumb is: *keep it simple.* Particularly with very young children, loading them down with complicated details can confuse the child. For children of any age, *let them know what to expect* and when—roughly—to expect it, particularly with obvious physical changes, such as the removal of your breast, hair loss, weight loss, and vomiting. Even young children can be told by giving them a simple, matter-of-fact explanation of *why* these changes are occurring: "Mommy's breast will need to be taken away by the doctor because there's something in it that's making her sick." If you can, make it humorous: "The medicine I'm taking makes me puke a lot, just like the dog when she eats grass!" "Yeah, the medicine makes me bald. Now I look just like Shaq!" If you can laugh about it, it will be less upsetting to them—and to you.

Obviously, you can't tell an infant or toddler what's up—they simply can't comprehend it. With such very young children, you need to communicate in nonverbal ways that they are important, which means taking time to play with them and spend time with them when your treatment schedule permits. Slightly older children (2 to 5 years old) can be told that Mommy is sick; you don't need to give them full medical details of your condition. It's enough for you to tell them that you're ill, that your doctor is taking care of you, and that for a while you might not be able to do some of the things you used to. But they, too, will need special time with you to reassure them that this sickness doesn't mean you're not going to

Telling your Children Keep it simple... let them know what to expect.

Changes Cancer Brings

be around any more. In school-age children six and older, you can give them even more information, depending on the child's level of comprehension. Use plain, simple language, and stay as close as possible to the truth. You'll likely need to tell them several times, not because they weren't listening or understanding, but because children often need repetition to make sure that what they've heard is "for real" and not a mistake or misunderstanding. Watch out for a child's natural tendency to assume that he or she is to blame for the illness—young children often assume that bad events are caused by something they did, said, or even thought, so it's a good idea to clearly explain to the child that your illness is unrelated to anything anyone might have done or said. Even when this "magical thinking" verges on the ridiculous—as in the story of the 7-year-old boy who thought the attack on the World Trade Center was a result of his poor grades in school—you should address it seriously: your child *really does believe that he or she is to blame for the catastrophe* and will need to be convinced that this is not the case.

Watch out for a child's natural tendency to assume that he or she is to blame.

Older children—14 years and up—should be given as much information as they request, though always with careful consideration of their emotional well-being and comprehension. Such information sharing is a sheer necessity because if they don't get the information from you, they're likely to go to another source—a library, a friend, a teacher, the Internet—and what they get from that source could cause them more stress than reassurance. If your teenager reads in a reference book that breast cancer is the second most frequent cause of death in women over 40, but you haven't told him or her that your diagnosis of DCIS has a 95% cure rate, your child will suffer greatly—and needlessly—from the misguided impression that your death is imminent. Don't try to force the details upon the child, however; tell him or her what is requested, and tell more only if you're asked for more. If there's difficulty in communicating with your teenager—not uncommon even when parents are healthy!—you can enlist the help of teachers, relatives, or friends to get the information across. If your teenager has difficulty coping with the diagnosis, you may consider family counseling to assist in working through the problems.

Even where adult children are concerned, many parents faced with this discussion simply don't know what to say or when to say it. The best time to open discussion on this topic is right after diagnosis is certain, before any treatments or hospitalization. As for what words to use, how much to say, when and where to tell them—that's something you need to determine, as the one who knows your child best. Fortunately, there are a few resources for parents who are looking for help in planning this talk. Online support groups, hotlines, local support groups, and anyone who has been through the experience can be helpful, so seek advice wherever you can. Cancer Care, Inc., offers a listing of such services, as does the American Cancer Society. Some books describing ways to tell young children about cancer, including books for children ages 2 to 10, are listed in the appendix.

83. My husband is divorcing me because I had a mastectomy. What can I do about that?

It's unfortunate, but true, that although serious illness or crisis brings some couples closer together, others are pushed apart. If you are confronted with the breakup of

Although serious illness or crisis brings some couples closer together, others are pushed apart.

your marriage at any point following your diagnosis, it's an added stress when you least need one—so don't try to deal with it alone. Contact a minister, a friend, or a counselor for advice. Unless your husband is adamant about ending your marriage—in which case it might simply be time to cut your losses, but more on that below—you might suggest marital counseling; it may be that whatever problem is causing him to want to end the marriage is something that can be resolved with professional assistance. Alternatively, suggest that instead of divorce, you try a separation for a while—perhaps until your treatment is over, or longer. It could be that all that's really required is a "breather" from the crisis, and given time, you and your husband can rebuild your marriage.

How you respond to the crisis in your marriage depends in large part on two factors: first, how much of an emotional investment do you have in this marriage? Second, what actions do you need to take to maintain both your emotional and physical well-being? If you have been married a long time and have a very close relationship, and if you feel that your partner is essential to your emotional well-being, then it may be worth spending some of your time and energy on rescuing your marriage rather than concentrating entirely on your treatment. Try to find out why he feels the marriage should end: it could simply be that he, as your primary caregiver, is feeling overwhelmed by his responsibilities and can find no other way to relieve this stress than by leaving your marriage. There are ways to relieve the admittedly intense stress of caregiving, and if this is what is causing the difficulty in an otherwise close, healthy relationship, you should help him seek out these methods. See Question 81 for more information on dealing with caregivers' problems.

Every relationship has its strains and stresses, which can become exposed during a crisis. Along with the shock of your diagnosis, you might also receive the shock of discovering that a relationship you thought was OK, isn't. Maybe the stress of being a caregiver isn't the cause of the breakup—maybe it's the last in a long line of reasons that simply went overlooked for too long. If this is the case and your husband is unwilling to work with you to salvage your marriage, you don't have much choice but to allow the divorce proceedings to go forward. It takes effort from two people, not one, to make a marriage work, and your top priority must be regaining your health. If this is the case, get an attorney and try to work something out that is quick and mutually acceptable to you both. Above all, make an effort to remain detached about the proceedings and to get as much emotional support as possible. Get it over with and move on to what's most important: your treatment and recovery.

Divorce doesn't mean your former husband can't continue to be a part of your life—he might even prove to be an invaluable source of support once relieved of the strain of an unhappy relationship. Some couples find that they're better friends once they've stopped being married. If, on the other hand, he wants nothing to do with you, then let him go. The anger, betrayal, and hurt you might feel are normal emotions, but don't wallow in them—they waste the energy you need to fight your cancer. There are plenty of people who will offer you what you need if he can't: support, affection, care, and even love. They may be relatives, friends, medical personnel, support group members, or even total strangers; the point is, if he can't give what you need, then look elsewhere for it. Don't spend your time and energy trying to get water from a stone.

84. What do I tell a young child (especially a girl) who sees my mastectomy?

If you live or work with young children, you can be certain that they will notice the change in your appearance and wonder about it. Even if you told the children in advance what was going to happen, they may not have comprehended that this would mean you would look different—a very young child might not understand that your earlier discussion about having your breast removed was "for real." Especially if the child is yours, he or she will want to know why the change occurred and be anxious about it, so you should prepare yourself to answer the child's questions (see Question 82).

With children, it's always best to keep it clear and simple, yet reassuring. If the child is openly curious as to why you have only one (or no) breast, you can tell her that the breast got sick and had to go to a special place to get better. If she wants to know whether it will come back, what you tell her depends on your plans. If you're planning a reconstruction, you can tell her that it will return—it's roughly the truth, and will satisfy her curiosity when you appear to have "gotten it back" following the reconstruction—but if not, your answer should be that it's going to stay in a place where someone can take good care of it while it's sick. It is important that you emphasize to the child that the absence of your breast is OK and appropriate, even if it's something you yourself are having difficulty accepting. You can do this by using a gentle but matter-of-fact tone in your voice, by keeping your voice low, by maintaining a relaxed posture, and by breathing slowly and deeply during the conversation—all subtle signals to the child that there is no danger or crisis involved in the discussion. It's not necessary to hide your emotions if you're sad over the loss of the breast—children understand sad feelings, and you can tell the child that you "miss" the breast, but that you will feel better in a little while because you know that its absence is OK. What the child does need to know, however, is that all is well and that the change in you does not indicate bigger, more frightening changes to come. Most of all, you should reassure the child that this sickness does not and will not affect *her*: a child's natural narcissism leads her to wonder if, because *you* got sick, that means *she'll* get sick too. Particularly with girls, who base much of their understanding of their feminine selves on the adult women in their lives, it's important to make sure they understand that this sickness in the breast is not something that need concern her (there is ample time to discuss her risk factors with her when she reaches adulthood). If she does show such concerns, you can play games of "Barbie goes to the doctor" with her dolls, directing the events so that Barbie comes out of the hospital alive, happy, and well.

Other children might not be as overt in their curiosity or might actually be frightened by your changed appearance. If this is the case, your response should again emphasize reassurance, not only that all is well with you, but that it's OK for them to approach you about it. One way of doing this is to discuss your mastectomy with another adult in the child's presence. Alternatively, you can broach the subject with the child herself, in a casual, nonconfrontational manner: "I don't know if you noticed it, but the doctor had to borrow a piece of my body for a little while. She did it to help me get better. I thought you should know that's what happened in case you were wondering." Follow up with an invitation for the child to ask questions anytime she wants to; she may not be ready to ask right away, but just knowing that it's OK to ask could alleviate some of her fears.

Just knowing that it's OK to ask could alleviate some of her fears.

PART SEVEN

The Impact of Cancer on Sexuality, Intimacy, and Fertility

How do my partner and I "deal" with
my mastectomy?

More . . .

85. How do my partner and I "deal" with my mastectomy?

A mastectomy can greatly affect a woman's body image and feelings of attractiveness (see Question 76) but it doesn't have to eliminate your sex life. You may need to do some experimentation and discussion with your partner to determine what is and what isn't comfortable for you, however. Some women who have had a mastectomy feel self-conscious being the partner on top during sex. The area of the missing breast is more visible in that position, so positions exposing her chest can make her feel vulnerable and insecure. For some, positions that put the woman's weight on her chest and shoulders can be painful, particularly if surgery extended to the lymph nodes under the arm. Such positions should be avoided, and supporting these areas with pillows during intercourse in other positions can help too.

If surgery removed only the tumor (segmental mastectomy or lumpectomy) and was followed by radiation therapy, the breast may still be scarred. It also may be different in shape or size. During the radiation period, the skin may become red and swollen. The breast also may be a little tender. Breast and nipple feeling, however, should remain normal.

Breast surgery or radiation to the breasts does not physically decrease a woman's sexual desire, nor does it affect her physiological responses during sex. Some good news from recent research is that most women with early-stage breast cancer have good emotional adjustment and sexual satisfaction by a year after their surgery. They report a quality of life similar to women who never had cancer.

86. How does a breast cancer diagnosis and treatment impact intimacy and sexuality?

The initial diagnosis can produce a great deal of anxiety and fear. How profound the anxiety and fear are varies depending on a woman's psychological health, lifestyle, and perception of her own sexuality. With the possibility of losing her breasts, a married woman or a woman who has a sexual partner might be concerned about her attractiveness. A single woman may be concerned about her ability to attract and satisfy a partner. One study stated that one year after a diagnosis of breast cancer up to 30% of women remain anxious, overwhelmingly distressed, and clinically depressed despite the treatment considerations.

Different treatments affect intimacy and sexuality in different ways. Surgical treatments, such as mastectomy and lumpectomy, can destroy nerves that provide stimulation to the nipples. Breast-conserving surgery (lumpectomy) provides no advantage over mastectomy in terms of sexual functioning and both have less of an impact on sexuality compared to nonsurgical treatment—radiation therapy, chemotherapy, hormonal therapy and the less studied immune therapy.

Radiation therapy is localized treatment and is well tolerated. Most damage is to the skin, causing redness, irritation, and possibly infection. Combined with decreased sensitivity of the breast, radiation therapy can affect stimulation or arousal.

Of the nonsurgical treatments, chemotherapy produces the greatest effect on sexual functioning because it alters hormone levels most. Even 5 to 10 years following chemotherapy treatment, some women report that they continue to experience sexual difficulties. Chemotherapy has many side effects. The most common are hair loss, nausea, vomiting, hot flashes, mouth sores, and weight gain. A more serious (but less obvious) side effect is decreased counts of various types of blood cells. Although an invisible side effect, decreased blood cell counts can have a significant impact on the patient's well-being: for example, decreases in white cells can increase the patient's susceptibility to infections. As with other types of cancer treatment, the type and severity of the side effects vary depending on which drugs are given, as well as the patient's overall health. After chemotherapy treatments are over, most side effects subside, and hair grows back. In premenopausal women, chemotherapy drugs *can* cause menstrual periods to halt, either temporarily or permanently.

Hormonal therapy works by affecting the way hormones in the body help cancers grow. It can be administered either by using drugs, such as tamoxifen, to block the action of these hormones, or by surgical removal of the ovaries. Some menopause-like effects can occur, but to a lesser degree than chemotherapy.

Targeted Biologic Therapy is the newest weapon in the fight against breast cancer and works by providing antibodies that are directed specifically against cancer cells. It is limited now to those cancers which are positive for the HER2 protein. The side effects are different to chemotherapy and include cardiac dysfunction and in rare case, heart failure.

87. Are there any medicines available that increase the desire for sex or make it more enjoyable? Compared to conventional treatments, are alternative medicines better at preserving sexuality?

Most women experience a decline in sex drive after breast cancer treatment, primarily as a result of chemotherapy. Chemotherapy causes the ovaries to stop producing estrogen as well as testosterone. Testosterone, although in small quantity, is partially responsible for sex drive. A hormone level can be drawn to determine if the level is low; however, testosterone replacement at this time is still controversial in breast cancer patients. There are no other prescription medications available to increase sex drive.

Jellies and creams can help combat dryness and improve sexual intercourse, so spread a small amount of water-soluble jelly on the outside of your vagina. Smart choices: K-Y jelly, Astroglide gel, Maxilube jelly, Replens pre-filled applicators, and Lubrin vaginal inserts.

(Do not start any self-treatments before checking with your doctor, so you can be sure any vaginal dryness or irritation is not due to an infection).

Alternative therapy

medicines used in lieu of standard medical therapies.

Complementary therapy

medicines used in conjunction with standard therapies.

Alternative therapy (medicines used in lieu of standard medical therapies) and **complementary therapy** (medicines used in conjunction with standard therapies) include a variety of herbal and food remedies, vitamins and other supplements, and traditional treatments such as acupuncture. Such therapies have become increasingly popular with the general public, and many are based upon traditional healing practices that have hundreds of years of use. Whether they actually work depends on the therapy you pick. Some alternative therapies are nothing more than scams taking advantage of patients' fears and longings for anything that will make the illness go away. They may do no harm—although some herbal agents can harm you. It is estimated that up to 30% of women use some form of alternative therapy either as a primary treatment or as a compliment to conventional treatment. Only a few studies have been conducted comparing both treatments, and no greater benefit is shown with alternative therapy versus conventional.

88. Because some concerns about diminished interest in sex are related to fatigue, are there any methods available to minimize fatigue during treatment?

Cancer patients often experience fatigue. It is a complicated side effect because there are many factors that contribute to feelings of tiredness. Sometimes it is the side effect of the chemotherapy drugs or radiation therapy. It can occur spontaneously in the absence of either of these adjuvant therapies. Yet resting—which seems the obvious solution to fatigue—sometimes does more harm than good: rest too much and your energy level actually decreases. Unlike most other symptoms, fatigue is the one side effect that often isn't treated medically but through adjustments in diet and lifestyle. The reasons for this are simple: fatigue is a symptom that comes and goes, that isn't predictable in onset or duration, and usually reflects the exertion of the body as it attempts to heal. Fatigue need not rule your life; you simply need to learn how to budget your energy to accomplish necessary tasks of day-to-day life. It may take a while to figure out how to pace yourself, but once you learn how much energy you have from day to day you can adjust your activities to accomplish the limits set by the healing process.

89. What methods are helpful in restoring intimacy after breast cancer treatment? When intimacy issues arise, where can I go for help?

Every woman and situation is unique. Being open-minded and willing to have open and honest conversations about your feelings is the best start. You and your partner may have concerns about pain after surgery. Trying to avoid the breast and exploring other areas for arousal can be exciting. Exploring your own body through self-touch can help increase your sensuality. If nervous about physical appearance from the loss of a breast or hair, wearing beautiful lingerie, dimming the lights, and listening to soothing music may help set the mood. Try being intimate at different times of day when energy levels are higher. There are also medications and herbal teas available that may reduce hot flashes and vaginal dryness.

Obviously a medical professional knowledgeable about intimacy, sexuality, and breast cancer issues may be the best source. However, your OB/GYN, oncology nurse, or other support staff may offer helpful information. A sex therapist or psychologist can offer methods to alleviate anxiety or fear that may be barriers to communication. A support group of women who are also dealing with breast cancer can help you discuss your feelings with others who have shared your experience.

90. Why is it that since my mastectomy I seem to be having difficulties with my partner—having sex less often and not enjoying it as much? Why am I afraid to let my partner get near me since my surgery?

Several studies have shown that some, but certainly not all, women who have had breast surgery may be faced with a problem involving their sexuality. There seem to be several parts to it, depending upon what kind of surgery you have had:

- You may be afraid of showing your scars to your partner.
- You may be afraid of having your partner see you with only one breast or with a breast that is not as perfect as before.
- You may feel you will never be the same person sexually as you were before.
- Your partner may be afraid of causing you pain.
- Your emotional problems may be more involved than having the breast operation.

For some, the loss is so great they cannot overcome it alone. If you are having a problem of this kind, it is important for you to seek professional help.

You may worry about the scar hurting or you may be afraid of letting your partner see your new body. Sexual relations can be resumed as soon as you feel ready. The body's ability to heal is quite rapid. Intimacy can help to make you feel better psychologically. A small, soft pillow to protect the scar may be helpful at first. You may need to experiment to find comfortable positions that do not put pressure on the area where you had surgery. Be honest with your partner. Explain your fears and enlist your partner's help. Your partner may also be afraid.

91. Are there other activities that will make me feel better about myself?

Physical exercise, such as tennis, swimming, dance classes, or exercise classes, can help to improve your feelings about yourself. Your sense of grace and balance can be enhanced through dance-exercise classes. Yoga has been recommended as a way of achieving a sense of wholeness about the body. Many persons have taken up challenging new activities, like skiing and rock climbing. Creative activities, such as music, painting, sewing, needlepoint, and writing, are excellent fields to explore to help strengthen your self-image. In addition, you may want to explore the possibility of breast reconstruction.

92. Are there factors unique to African-American women that may affect their sexuality?

Most women are concerned about body appearance after surgery, but African-American women have a greater chance of **keloid formation** (smooth, thick elevated scars that can develop after the skin is traumatized by a cut, burn, or other injury)—a dermatological nuisance. If you are prone to keloiding, make certain you tell your surgeon. The doctor may be able to prevent keloids from forming by injecting an anti-inflammatory steroid medicine at the incision site during or following surgery. Hair loss and damage are also issues of concern for African-American women. Chemical relaxers, weaves,

Keloid formation

smooth, thick, elevated scars that can develop after the skin is traumatized by a cut, burn, or other injury.

and coloring the hair should be minimized. Weight and size comparisons have been the bane of African-American women. In American culture, weight and size is generally associated with being unattractive, creating a breeding ground for negative images of African-American women. African-American women have denser bones and thicker skin and hips, and in African-American culture, a heftier figure is viewed as a sign of good health and fertility. A healthy body weight coupled with diet and exercise is essential for all women. African-American women, however, typically have a healthier outlook about their body image.

93.   If I'm pregnant when I'm diagnosed, should I delay treatment so it won't affect my baby? What if I get pregnant while I'm getting radiation or chemotherapy?

Although breast cancer is more common in post-menopausal women, it is far from rare in women of childbearing age. Thus, it does sometimes occur in women who are pregnant, and with many women delaying childbearing until they are in their 30s and early 40s, the incidence of breast cancer coinciding with pregnancy is rising. Currently, about 1 in 3000 pregnant or lactating women will develop breast cancer.

Diagnosis of cancer in a pregnant or lactating woman is complicated by the fact that standard diagnostic tools sometimes can't be used. The changes to the breast associated with pregnancy tend to interfere with the detection of lumps and similar symptoms, so the signals that normally alert a woman to the possibility of disease may go overlooked or disregarded. Even when such signals are noted, the usual follow-up procedure—a mammogram—is sometimes delayed out of fear for the safety of the fetus. Although the National Cancer Institute, M.D. Anderson Cancer Center, and other prominent information sources state that standard mammography does not harm the fetus if proper shielding is used, most physicians—and their patients—are reluctant to risk giving the fetus even minimal exposure to radiation, and so avoid mammography. For this reason, it is common for pregnant or lactating women to be diagnosed at a more advanced stage of cancer.

Research has shown that once a woman has been diagnosed with breast cancer during pregnancy, her chances of survival are less than a nonpregnant woman, for every stage. This may be even more serious for African-American women who already have more aggressive cancers and poorer prognoses, independent of pregnancy. Termination of pregnancy has not been shown to improve survival. Women who are at high risk, particularly those with a family history, may want to be screened for breast cancer *before* trying to conceive.

Strategies for treatment of breast cancer in pregnant women are determined by two factors: the stage of the fetus' development, and the stage of the cancer. In the first trimester of pregnancy, radiation and chemotherapy cannot be administered because both will cause damage to the fetus, so mastectomy is usually recommended over breast-conserving therapies for women with early stage cancers (stage I and II). After the first trimester, some chemotherapy regimens can be used without fearing deformities or damage to the baby, although low birth weight is a concern. Radiation therapy, however, is harmful to the fetus at any stage of development and should be postponed until after the baby is born.

Women with later stage cancers—those typically treated aggressively with radiation and chemotherapy after surgery—face a difficult decision. They can choose to delay treatment until the baby is born, which creates the risk that their cancer will advance far enough to become a grave threat to their own lives. They can wait until the first trimester has passed, then embark upon a chemotherapy regimen that is not aggressive enough to impact the baby, but that may also be less effective against the cancer. Alternatively, they can end the pregnancy through an induced abortion and proceed with aggressive radiation and chemotherapy treatments, although this option is generally suggested only to those women still in the first trimester. Abortion in and of itself does not improve the woman's prognosis; all it does is permit the use of more aggressive chemotherapy and radiation therapy, which could save her life if her cancer is far advanced. Many women find the idea of ending a pregnancy for any reason unacceptable from an emotional, moral, or religious standpoint, and it's important to know that you don't *have* to do it—but you need to accept the fact that, if you decide to continue your pregnancy, some of the more effective treatment strategies may not be available to you. It's generally wise to consult with family members, counselors, or close friends when faced with this decision—above all, make sure you have plenty of emotional support. Ultimately, it is the patient's decision, not the doctor's or anyone else's, whether or not to end a pregnancy in order to select more aggressive treatment for the cancer.

94. Can I have children and breast-feed after my treatment for cancer is finished? Will pregnancy cause a recurrence of breast cancer? When is it safe for a woman to become pregnant after breast cancer?

It is not unusual for women who have had breast cancer to subsequently have children, and some are even able to breast-feed their babies with the treated breast. This end result requires careful planning in the surgery and adjuvant therapy chosen to treat the cancer—and a little bit of luck, since maintaining the structures needed for breast-feeding through surgical treatment can be difficult at best. The possibility of retaining your fertility and your ability to breast-feed depends in large part upon your diagnosis and the particulars of your tumor: small, early-stage tumors have the most potential for a good outcome, but the larger the tumor and later the stage, the lower your chances for this result.

Surgery is the first line of treatment for pregnant women with breast cancer. Women with later stage cancers—those typically treated aggressively with radiation and chemotherapy after surgery—face a difficult decision. They can choose to delay treatment until the baby is born, which creates the risk that their cancer will advance far enough to become a grave threat to their own lives. Women with earlier-stage cancer can wait until the first trimester has passed, then embark upon a chemotherapy regimen that is not aggressive enough to impact the baby, but that may also be less effective against the cancer. Many women find the idea of ending a pregnancy for any reason unacceptable from an emotional, moral, or religious standpoint, and it's important to know that you don't have to do it—but you need to accept the fact that, if you decide to continue your pregnancy, some of the more effective treatment strategies may not be available to you. It's generally wise to consult with family members, counselors, or close friends when faced with this decision—above all, make sure you have plenty of emotional support. Ultimately, it is the patient's decision, not the doctor's or anyone else's, whether to end a pregnancy in order to select more aggressive treatment for cancer.

A recent study showed no increase in cancer recurrences for women who became pregnant after breast cancer. For the few women who did have a recurrence, however, that recurrence happened faster if they became pregnant. Because pregnancy raises estrogen levels in the body, it is important for women to discuss their individual medical history and the safety of pregnancy with their doctors. Women are usually advised to wait two to five years (disease free) after the completion of treatment to become pregnant. (The first five years is the most likely time for a recurrence.) Women should also discuss the impact of pregnancy on their general health, as chemotherapy can sometimes cause undetected damage to the heart and lungs.

Studies show that children born to cancer survivors after cancer treatment appear to have no more birth defects than children born into the general population. In addition, they have no greater risk for developing cancer, except in rare cases of truly genetic cancers.

In many women, cancer treatment causes menstruation to stop temporarily. This is a normal bodily response to a high degree of stress—a way of conserving bodily resources for the high-priority task of healing, rather than expending them unnecessarily on reproduction. Most of the time, menstrual cycles resume within a few months of the end of treatment, but there is no absolute guarantee that this will occur: you might find your menstrual cycles come less frequently, that you sometimes skip one or more periods, or even that they don't come back at all. Both radiation and chemotherapy can affect fertility permanently, particularly if you're already over 40 and approaching the normal age for menopause. Some chemotherapy regimens actually cause premature menopause, so if you had been considering having children prior to your cancer diagnosis, make sure your oncologist is aware of this fact prior to undergoing any sort of treatment—if he or she knows that fertility is a concern, the oncologist is more likely to choose strategies to improve the chances that you'll avoid premature menopause.

With respect to potential impacts on your ovaries, chemotherapy only impacts the menstrual cycle—it doesn't affect the eggs themselves, because they aren't dividing cells, so the drugs don't act on them. Certain radiation therapies, particularly implant radiation, might adversely affect the ova (eggs), however. If your cancer is advanced enough to require very aggressive therapies, you might consider consulting with a fertility specialist prior to beginning treatment; such specialists might be able to offer strategies to either minimize the impact of radiation therapy on your reproductive system or counteract its effects following treatment. One possibility is to have ova extracted from your ovaries prior to treatment, fertilized in vitro, and frozen to await implantation after your treatment is done. This method prevents your reproductive tissue from sustaining damage during treatment, and it also allows you to give birth even if your ovaries do shut down permanently because of the chemotherapy regimen you're on—but it can be extremely expensive, and it's hardly ever covered by insurance.

As noted earlier, many doctors suggest a waiting period of two to five years following treatment for breast cancer before you get pregnant. Because most signs of recurrence occur within this time, waiting allows you to be reasonably certain of your health prior to beginning a pregnancy. This is particularly important if your cancer was hormone sensitive, as recurrent cancer could be exacerbated by the hormone increases associated with pregnancy. If you don't feel you can wait that long because of your age, you should at minimum wait a year or so to give your body time to recover from the effects of chemotherapy before subjecting it to the stresses of pregnancy.

Depending on the extent of your tumor and the treatment strategies chosen, you may be able to retain your ability to have children but lose your ability to breast-feed. This effect might only be temporary: in women who are diagnosed during or immediately after their pregnancy, for example, adjuvant chemotherapy requires that infants be weaned to a bottle, because the drugs used in treatment will pass through the breast milk into the baby and are likely to be harmful, but in theory any subsequent children the patient might have would still be able to breast-feed from that breast, assuming surgical treatment has left the structures intact. However, extensive surgery and radiation therapy could damage the lobules and ducts enough to permanently prevent breast-feeding from the affected breast. If this were the case, you'd still have the unaffected breast for this purpose; the only problem is that your breasts will likely become asymmetrical in size because the healthy breast will grow in response to milk production, but the treated breast will not. You can, however, have breast-reduction surgery once you're done having and feeding babies.

If your future ability to breast-feed is important to you, bring up the subject to your surgeon and your oncologist before undergoing any treatment. Although they might not be able to do anything about it—after all, the top priority is ridding your body of the cancer, and breast-feeding is a secondary concern—if you let them know this is important to you, they'll do the best they can.

95. What breast cancer treatments put women's fertility at risk and why? If a woman is not in menopause after treatment, has her fertility been affected?

Chemotherapy presents the main risk to a patient's fertility. Breast cancer patients usually receive either CMF (cyclophospamide, methotezate, and 5-flurouracil); or AC (adriamycin and cyclophosphamide). Cyclophosphamide (Cytoxan) is known to have a negative affect on ovarian function. Women receiving cyclophosphamide are four times more likely to develop ovarian failure, compared with controls. The chance of immediate ovarian failure increases with age and for CMF it is 78% and for AC it is 38% (for a 40-year-old breast cancer patient).

Radiation and surgery can also impact a patient's fertility, if they affect the reproductive organs. However, this is not generally the case for most breast cancer patients.

Since each course of chemotherapy will result in the loss of a significant portion of ovarian reserve, even those who do not immediately become menopausal following chemotherapy are likely to experience early menopause. In addition, as previously noted, many experts do not recommend pregnancy for at least two to five years (recurrence free) after breast cancer diagnosis and treatment. During this interval, many patients who are not immediately infertile after chemotherapy will become infertile due to their diminished ovarian reserve and natural aging. Patients should work closely with their doctors to discuss these issues.

96. What options exist to preserve fertility for women with breast cancer? Are these options safe?

Several treatments are available for women to preserve their fertility. The availability and efficacy of these treatments varies based on a number of biomedical and social factors. Some of these options are well established, while others are experimental. Factors such as cost, partner status, the patient's age, and diagnosis may influence the choice of an option.

- **Embryo freezing** is the most established method of preserving a woman's fertility. Hormones are used to mature a woman's eggs, which are then removed and fertilized by in vitro fertilization (IVF). Embryos are then frozen for future use. This process requires sperm provided by a husband or partner. Donor sperm can also be used. All of the steps required to freeze embryos take about two to six weeks, depending on the type of stimulation used.

- **Egg freezing** is an experimental option which may be attractive to single women who do not have a male partner and do not want to use donor sperm. Although egg freezing pregnancy rates are lower than embryo freezing, the techniques are improving rapidly. For the woman, the steps required to freeze eggs are the same as those required to freeze embryos, and they take about two to six weeks.

- **Ovarian tissue freezing** may be a good option when there is little or no time for ovarian stimulation before treatment. Tissue from the ovary is removed, cryopreserved (frozen), and then reimplanted later. Ovarian tissue freezing is still experimental. Some tissue transplants have been successful and have caused women to resume hormonal functioning, but there has been only one birth to date.

- **Gonadotropin-releasing hormone analog (GnRH-a)** treatment is an experimental treatment that is sometimes offered during chemotherapy treatment. It is thought to protect ovarian function by temporarily putting the ovaries into a dormant state. More research is needed to determine whether GnRH-a treatment is safe and effective.

Some fertility preservation options such as embryo freezing and egg freezing require hormone stimulation.

The hormones used can raise a women's estrogen level, which can be a concern for breast cancer patients, especially those who are ER positive. There are, however, some techniques that can be used such as tamoxifen-IVF or Letrozole stimulation, that may be safer for breast cancer patients. In addition, many oncologists feel that one round of stimulation *before* chemotherapy is acceptable. Patients need to discuss these risks and benefits with their doctor to understand which option is safe for them.

97. What is the average cost of fertility-preserving treatments? How do women with limited resources (e.g., financial and social support) gain access to these services?

The cost of fertility preservation can be high and is usually not covered by health insurance. The average cost of egg and embryo freezing is $8000 to $10,000 (not including drugs). Ovarian tissue freezing is approximately $12,000. The costs of adoption, however, can also be high, and depending on the type of adoption involved can range from $2500 to $35,000.

It is difficult for women with limited financial resources to access these services. Some insurance companies do cover some of the costs involved. Some patients are also able to work with their infertility team and/or pharmaceutical companies involved to get a discount on the drugs or services needed. Fertile Hope (a nonprofit organization dedicated to helping people with cancer who are faced with infertility; www. fertile.org or call

888-994-HOPE) has launched Sharing Hope, the first financial assistance program for cancer patients who want to preserve their fertility.

98. What fertility treatments are available for women who have already completed treatment and who may be moving towards early menopause?

Women who remain fertile after completing chemotherapy may want to consider preserving their fertility if they are not yet ready to start a family but are concerned about having children in the future. Because it is impossible to know when early menopause might occur, some women choose to freeze embryos, eggs, or ovarian tissue after treatment.

99. What are the options for women who are infertile after treatment?

- **Donor eggs** and **donor embryos** are an option for women who go into early menopause after treatment. These options allow a woman to become pregnant and carry a child; and, in the case of donor eggs, that child could have a biological connection to the woman's partner.
- **Surrogacy** is when another woman carries a child for you. This may be a choice for a woman if her doctor believes that pregnancy after breast cancer is not safe, or if she is unable to carry a pregnancy.
- **Adoption** can be an excellent way to become a parent. Adoption can be private or public, domestic or international. Adoption agencies may look at your medical history, so it is a good idea to select an agency that is open to working with cancer survivors.

100. Where can I go to find more information?

The information in this book barely scratches the surface of what's available to breast cancer patients and their families. The accompanying appendix offers a selection of good resources to address many topics.

The Impact of Cancer on Sexuality

Appendix

Organizations

American Academy of Medical Acupuncture
www.medicalacupuncture.org
(323) 937–5514
AAMA, 4929 Wilshire Boulevard, Suite 428, Los Angeles, CA 90010

American Cancer Society
www.cancer.org
1–800–ACS–2345
American Cancer Society National Home Office, 1599 Clifton Road, Atlanta,
   GA 30329

American Society of Clinical Oncology
www.asco.org
703–299–0150
1900 Duke Street, Suite 200, Alexandria, VA 22314

Avon Breast Cancer Foundation
www.avoncrusade.com
Avon Breast Cancer Crusade, 1345 Avenue of the Americas, New York, NY
   10105

Breastcancer.org
www. breastcancer.org
(An online nonprofit organization)

The Breast Cancer Resource Committee
www.bcresource.org
202–261–3518 / 202–261–3508 fax
2121 K Street NW, Washington, DC 20037

Breast Cancer Society of Canada
www.bcsc.ca
800–567–8767
401 St. Clair Street, Point Edward, ON, Canada N7V 1P2

Canadian Breast Cancer Network
www.cbcn.ca
613–230–3044
Toll Free: 1–800–685–8820
Suite 602, 331 Cooper Street, Ottawa, ON, Canada, K2P 0G5

Cancer Care, Inc.
www.cancercare.org
212–712–8400 (admin); 212–712–8080 (services)
275 7th Avenue, New York, NY 10001

Cancer Research Institute
www.cancerresearch.org
1–800–99–CANCER (800–992–2623)
681 Fifth Avenue, New York, NY 10022

Centers for Disease Control and Prevention
www.cdc.gov
(404) 639–3534
Toll Free: 1–800–311–3435
1600 Clifton Road, Atlanta, GA 30333

Department of Veterans Affairs
www.va.gov
202–273–5400 (Washington, D.C., office)
Toll Free: 1–800–827–1000 (reaches local VA office)
Veterans Health Association, 810 Vermont Avenue NW, Washington, DC 20420

Health Insurance Association of America
www.hiaa.org
202–824–1600
555 13th Street NW, Suite 600, East Washington, DC
20004–1109

Health Resources and Services Administration
Hill-Burton Program
www.hrsa.gov/osp/dfcr/about/aboutdiv.htm
301–443–5656
Toll Free: 1–800–638–0742 / 1–800–492–0359 (if calling from
the Maryland area)
Health Resources and Services Administration, U.S. Department
of Health and Human Services, Parklawn Building, 5600 Fish-
ers Lane, Rockville, MD 20857

Institute of Certified Financial Planners
www.icfp.org
303–759–4900
Toll Free: 1–800–282–7526 (automated referral service)

Living Beyond Breast Cancer
www.lbbc.org
610–645–4567
10 East Athens Avenue, Suite 204, Ardmore, PA 19003

National Breast Cancer Coalition
www.natlbcc.org
800–622–2838
1101 17th Street, N.W., Suite 1300, Washington, DC 20036
202–296–7477 / 202–265–6854 fax

National Cancer Institute
www.nci.nih.gov
301–435–3848 (Public Information Office line).
National Cancer Institute Public Information Office, Building
31, Room 10A31, 31 Center Drive, MSC 2580, Bethesda,
MD 20892–2580

Appendix

National Center for Complementary and Alternative Medicine
nccam.nih.gov
1–888–644–6226
NCCAM Clearinghouse, P.O. Box 7923, Gaithersburg, MD
20898

National Comprehensive Cancer Network
www.nccn.org
888–909–NCCN (888–909–6226)
50 Huntingdon Pike, Suite 200, Rockledge, PA 19046

National Lymphedema Network
www.lymphnet.org
1–800–541–3259
Latham Square, 1611 Telegraph Avenue, Suite 1111, Oakland,
CA 94612–2138

National Viatical Association
www.nationalviatical.org
202–429–5129
Toll free: 1–800–741–9465
Viatical Association of America, 1200 Nineteenth Street, NW,
Washington, DC 20036–2412

Sisters Network, Inc.
www.sistersnetwork.org
866-781-1808

Social Security Administration
Office of Public Inquiries
http://www.ssa.gov/
Toll Free Number: 1–(800) 772–1213 / 1–(800) 325–0778
(TTY)
Social Security Administration, Office of Public Inquiries, 6401
Security Blvd., Room 4-C–5 Annex, Baltimore, MD
21235–6401

SusanLoveMD.com
www.susanlovemd.com
310–230–1712
Box 846, Pacific Palisades, CA 90272

The Susan G. Komen Foundation
www.komen.org
800-IM AWARE (800–462–9273)
5005 LBJ Freeway, Suite 250, Dallas, TX 75244

United Seniors Health Cooperative
www.unitedseniorshealth.org
202–479–6973
Toll Free: 1–800–637–2604
USHC, Suite 200, 409 Third Street SW, Washington, DC
    20024

Y-ME National Breast Cancer Organization
www.y-me.org
800–221–2141
212 W. Van Buren, Suite 500, Chicago, IL 60607

Web Sites with General Cancer Information

- 411Cancer.com
- About.com (search on "cancer")
- BCDG.org
- Breast Cancer Answers/University of Wisconsin Comprehensive Cancer Center, www.medsch.wisc.edu/bca/bca.html
- CancerLinks.org
- CancerSource.com
- CancerWiseTM / MD Anderson Cancer Center, www.cancerwise.org
- National Cancer Institute's CancerNet Service, cancernet.nci.nih.gov/index.html
- TheBreastClinic.com
- WCN.org
- www.medsch.wisc.edu/bca/link.htm
- YWCA.org/html/B4d1.asp

Web Pages on Specific Cancer Topics

Alternative Therapy
Information on acupuncture: www.medicalacupuncture.org (see American Academy for Medical Acupuncture).

Comprehensive Web site about alternative therapies for cancer: www.healthy.net/asp/templates/center.asp?centerid=23.

Breast Reconstruction

The American Society of Plastic and Reconstructive Surgeons and Plastic Surgery Educational Foundation offer a site (www.plasticsurgery.org/surgery/brstrec.htm) about the process of breast reconstruction.

www.breastdiseases.com/pe11.htm explains the different types of breast reconstruction and procedures.

Chemotherapy

www.yana.org offers online and in-person support groups for those going through high-dose chemotherapy.

Drug information for chemotherapy and hormonal therapy, including information on financial assistance: www.cancersupportivecare.com/pharmacy.html.

Clinical Trials

National Cancer Institute's CancerTrials site lists current clinical trials that have been reviewed by NCI: cancertrials.nci.nih.gov.

Coping

National Coalition for Cancer Survivorship (www.cansearch.org, 1–877–NCCS–YES) offers a free audio program, *Cancer Survivor Toolbox*, including ways to cope with the illness. (Web site also has a newsletter, requiring yearly membership fee.)

R. A. Bloch Cancer Foundation (www.blochcancer.org) offers an inspirational online book about cancer, relaxation techniques, and positive outlooks on fighting cancer, as well as trained one-on-one support from fellow cancer patients.

Diet and Nutrition (Cancer Prevention)

USDA Dietary Guidelines: www.mypyramid.gov.

American Institute for Cancer Research provides tips on how to reduce cancer risk at www.aicr.org.

Cancer Research Foundation of America's Healthy Eating Suggestions: www.preventcancer.org/whdiet.cfm.

Family Resources

www.kidscope.org is a Web site designed to help children understand and deal with the effects of cancer on a parent.

Men's Crusade Against Breast Cancer
(home.earthlink.net/~rkupbens/mcabc) is a resource for husbands and other family members, providing support, ways to cope, and promotion of research.

Genetic Counseling

The National Society of Genetic Counselors Web site (www.nsgc.org) lists society members, complete with specialty.

The National Cancer Institute has a searchable list of health care professionals who specialize in genetics and can provide information and counseling at www.cancernet.nci.nih.gov/genesrch.shtml.

Case study on breast cancer and genetic counseling: www.intouchlive.com/home/frames.htm? www.intouchlive.com/cancergenetics/index.htm&3

Articles on genetics and cancer: cancer.med.upenn.edu/causeprevent/genetics/.

Hair Loss

Look Good, Feel Better program through local American Cancer Society offices or at 1–800–395–LOOK.

A full-color catalogue of wigs for medical purposes is available nationwide. Contact Jacques Darcel, 50 West 57th Street, New York, NY 10019, 212-753–7576.

Buyer's Guide to Wigs and Hairpieces. This 2-page summary is available, as well as additional literature as needed. Contact Ruth L. Weintraub Co. Inc., 420 Madison Avenue, Suite 406, New York, NY 10017, 212-838–1333.

HER2 Gene

www.herceptin.com is a web site by the makers of Herceptin that contains information about the HER2 gene and its connection to breast cancer. A second site, www.her2support.org, is maintained by an independent patient-support organization called HER2 Support Group.

Hormonal Therapy

National Cancer Institute's fact sheet "Questions and Answers about Tamoxifen": cis.nci.nih.gov/fact/7_16.htm; also, "Understanding Estrogen Receptors, Tamoxifen, and Raloxifene", rex.nci.nih.gov/behindthenews/uest/uestframe.htm.

Frequently asked questions about tamoxifen: www.cancersupportivecare.com/tamoxifen.html.

Inflammatory Breast Cancer

IBC Help and Support page: www.bestiary.com/ibc

Inflammatory Breast Cancer Research Foundation, http://www.ibcresearch.org

IBC Research Foundation, P.O. Box 90117, Anchorage, AK 99509

Legal Protections, Financial Resources, and Insurance Coverage

The American Cancer Society offers a number of relevant documents to help understand your coverage, legal protections, and how to find financial assistance. Search www.cancer.org using keyword "insurance."

Medicaid Information: www.hcfa.gov/medical/medicaid.htm

"Every Question You Need to Ask Before Selling Your Life Insurance Policy."

National Viator Representatives, Inc. Call 1–800–932–0050 for a free copy. www.nvrnvr.com.

Family and Medical Leave Act: www.dol.gov/dol/esa/public/regs/statutes/whd/fmla.htm.

Health Care Financing Administration's (HCFA) Web site about Breast Cancer and Medicaid programs: www.hcfa.gov/medicaid/bccpt/default.htm.

www.needymeds.com offers information about programs sponsored by pharmaceutical manufacturers to help people who cannot afford to purchase necessary drugs.

www.cancercare.org/hhrd/hhrd_financial.htm offers listings of where to look for financial assistance.

The National Financial Resource Book for Patients: A State-by-State Directory: data.patientadvocate.org.

Lymphedema

National Lymphedema Network, www.lymphnet.org.

Mammography Information

American College of Radiology/Radiological Society of North America gives a detailed discussion of what mammography is, step-by-step explanation of the procedure, and pictures of the equipment, answering questions about the safety and comfort of the procedure: www.radiologyinfo.org/content/mammogram.htm.

Informational page including frequently asked questions about mammograms: www.cancercare.org/types/breast/detection.asp.

Male Breast Cancer

About Male Breast Cancer,
interact.withus.com/interact/mbc/about.htm.

The Susan G. Komen Foundation: Male Breast Cancer,
www.breastcancerinfo.com/bhealth/html/male_breast_cancer.asp.

www.menagainstbreastcancer.org

Metastatic Breast Cancer

Resource center solely for patients with metastatic breast cancer: www.patientcenters.com/breastcancer

Minorities and Breast Cancer

The Breast Cancer Resource Committee seeks to educate African-American women about breast cancer: www.resource.org

National Asian Women's Health Organization

www.nawho.org/womens_health/bcc_program.html
1–415–989–9747
250 Montgomery Street, Suite 900, San Francisco CA, 94104.

The Living Beyond Breast Cancer Foundation

(www.lbbc.org/outreach.asp) offers a complimentary book specifically for African-American women: *Getting Connected: African Americans Living Beyond Breast Cancer.*

www.cancerlinks.org/breast.html#ETHNIC offers a listing of breast cancer websites for different ethnic groups.

www.blackwomenshealth.com has a section on dealing with breast cancer.

Myths about Breast Cancer

General information on breast cancer myths:
www.imaginis.com/breasthealth/bcmyths.asp or www.cancer-wise.org/facts_figures/ff_breast.html.

Specific debunking of the antiperspirant myth:
www.pathguy.com/antipers.htm.

Nausea/Vomiting

National Comprehensive Cancer Network:
www.nccn.org/patient_guidelines/nausea-and-vomiting/nausea-and-vomiting/1_introduction.htm.

Royal Marsden Hospital Patient Information On Line:
www.royalmarsden.org/patientinfo/booklets/coping/nausea7.asp#heading.

Treatment Locators: Physicians and Hospitals

AIM DocFinder (state medical board executive directors): www.docboard.org.
Nonprofit organization providing a health professional licensing database.

AMA Physician Select (American Medical Association):
www.ama-assn.org/aps/amahg.htm. AMA database of demographic and professional information on individual physicians in the United States.

American Board of Medical Specialties: Provides verification of physician qualifications and has lists of specialists.
www.abms.org, 1–866-ASK-ABMS or American Board of Medical Specialties, 1007 Church Street, Suite 404, Evanston, IL 60201–5913.

BreastDoctor.com: www.breastdoctor.com
Access to a physician directory focused on breast cancer.

Health Check: The 318 Top Cancer Specialists for Women
(Good Housekeeping):
goodhousekeeping.women.com/gh/eatwell/health/tools/39docs16.htm.
Lists the leading clinicians for lung, breast, and colon cancer in women as found in a survey of department chairs and section chiefs at major U.S. medical centers. Breast cancer specialists (surgical, medical, and radiation oncologists) may be searched

geographically. The list appeared in the March 1999 issue of *Good Housekeeping*.

Best Hospitals Finder *(U.S. News & World Report)*:
www.usnews.com/usnews/nycu/health/hosptl/tophosp.htm.
The *U.S. News* hospital rankings are designed to assist patients in their search for the highest level of medical care. Database is searchable by specialty, including the top cancer hospitals (www.usnews.com/usnews/nycu/health/hosptl/speccanc.htm) or by geographic region.

Best HMOs Finder *(U.S. News & World Report)*:
www.usnews.com/usnews/nycu/health/hetophmo.htm.
U.S. News guide to choosing a managed-care option.

Hospital Select (American Medical Association & Medical-Net, Inc.):
www.hospitalselect.com/curb_db/owa/sp_hospselect.main.
Hospital locator database searchable by hospital name, city, state, or zip code. Hospital Select data include basic information (name, address, telephone number); beds and utilization; service lines; and accreditation.

HospitalWeb (Dept. of Neurology, Massachusetts General Hospital):
neuro-www.mgh.harvard.edu/hospitalweb.shtml.
Searchable database of hospital Web sites.

National Cancer Institute Designated Cancer Centers: cancertrials.nci.nih.gov/finding/centers/html/map.html.
Directory of NCI-designated Cancer Centers, 58 research-oriented U.S. institutions recognized for scientific excellence and extensive cancer resources. Listings feature phone contact numbers, Web site links and a brief summary of Web site resources.

National Comprehensive Cancer Network (NCCN):
www.nccn.org.
The National Comprehensive Cancer Network (NCCN) is an alliance of leading cancer centers. NCCN members (www.nccn.org/profiles.htm) provide the highest quality in cancer care and cancer research. NCCN offers a patient information and referral service (www.nccn.org/newsletters/1999_may/ page_5.htm) that

responds to cancer-related inquiries and provides referrals to member institutions' programs and services (1–888–909–6226).

Approved Hospital Cancer Program *(Commission on Cancer of the American College of Surgeons)*: www.facs.org/public_info/yourhealth/aahcp.html. The Approvals Program of the Commission on Cancer surveys hospitals, treatment centers, and other facilities according to standards set by the Committee on Approvals which recommends approval awards in specific categories based on these surveys. A hospital that has received approval has voluntarily committed itself to providing the best in diagnosis and treatment of cancer. Approved hospitals can be searched by city, state, and category.

Association of Community Cancer Centers: Cancer Centers and Member Profiles: www.accc-cancer.org/members/map.html. Geographic listing of ACCC members with contact information, and description of cancer program and services *as provided by the member institutions.*

HMOs and other managed care plans *(Cancer care)*: www.cancercare.org/patients/hmos.htm. Discusses the advantages and disadvantages of HMO care.

Paget's Disease
The Paget Foundation's home page: www.paget.org.

Physician Qualifications
The American Board of Medical Specialities: www.abms.org; click the "who's certified" button (search by physician name or by specialty).

Pregnancy
The National Cancer Institute (CancerNet) has up-to-date information dealing with pregnancy and breast cancer, including treatment options, information about breast-feeding, etc: www.cancernet.nci.nih.gov/cgibin/srchcgi.exe?DBID=pdq&TYPE=search&SFMT=pdq_statement/1/0/0&Z208=208_05380P.

MD Anderson Cancer Center has a protocol regarding pregnancy and breast cancer: www.mdanderson.org/diseases/breastcancer/pregnancy.

Radiation Therapy

National Cancer Institute/CancerNet: Radiation Therapy and You: A Guide to Self-Help During Cancer Treatment cancernet.nci.nih.gov/peb/radiation. By phone, free of charge: 1–800–4–CANCER (in English and Spanish).

Research Updates

The BreastCancer.net Web site features up-to-date news about breast cancer research and treatments: www.breastcancer.net/bcn.html.

Risk Assessment

National Cancer Institute's Risk Assessment Tool on CancerNet, cancernet.nci.nih.gov/bcra_tool.html.

Sexuality and Breast Cancer

Effects of breast cancer and treatment on sexuality and ways to cope: www.cancercare.org/campaigns/breast1.htm.

Support Groups

National Alliance of Breast Cancer Organization listing of support groups by state: www.nabco.org/support.

Cancer Hope Network provides free one-on-one support for cancer patients and their families by volunteers who've been through the cancer experience (www.cancerhopenetwork.org/, 1–877–HOPENET).

Association of Cancer Online Resources provides an online Breast Cancer support group: listserv.acor.org/archives/BRCA.html.

The Wellness Community (www.wellness-community.org, 1–888–793–WELL) provides support groups, educational workshops, social events, etc. for cancer patients and their families at its facilities around the country.

Surgical Treatment

www.breastdiseases.com/pe8.htm offers explanations of the different types of surgery as well as advantages and disadvantages of each.

http://cancerconsultants.onco-web.com/RxOverview/Breast-Overview/Surgery.htm gives an overview of breast cancer surgery, as well as detailed explanations of the different kinds of surgery.

Terminology

Glossary of Breast Cancer Terms: www.cancerhelp.com/ed/ glossary.htm.

Breast Cancer Glossary: breastcancer.about.com/library/ glossary/blglossar.htm?terms=breast+cancer.

Books and Pamphlets

The following books are available from the American Cancer Society:

- *The American Cancer Society's Guide to Pain Control: Powerful Methods to Overcome Cancer Pain*
- *Coming to Terms with Cancer*
- *Informed Decisions, 2nd Edition*
- *American Cancer Society's Guide to Complementary and Alternative Cancer Methods*
- *Caregiving*
- *Women and Cancer*
- *A Breast Cancer Journey*

The following pamphlets are available from the National Cancer Institute:

- *Chemotherapy and You: A Guide to Self-Help During Treatment*
- *Eating Hints for Cancer Patients Before, During, and After Treatment*
- *Get Relief From Cancer Pain*
- *Helping Yourself During Chemotherapy*
- *Questions and Answers About Pain Control: A Guide for People with Cancer and Their Families*
- *Taking Time: Support for People With Cancer and the People Who Care About Them*
- *Taking Part in Clinical Trials: What Cancer Patients Need to Know*

Available in Spanish:
- *Datos sobre el tratamiento de quimioterapia contra el cancer*
- *El tratamiento de radioterapia; guia para el paciente durante el tratamiento*
- *En que consisten los estudios clinicos? Un folleto para los pacientes de cancer*

The following pamphlets are available from the National Comprehensive Cancer Network:
- *Breast Cancer Treatment Guidelines for Patients*
- *Cancer Pain Treatment Guidelines for Patients*
- *Nausea and Vomiting Treatment Guidelines for Patient with Cancer*

Available in Spanish:
- *Cáncer de seno*
- *El dolor asociado con el cáncer*

Helpful Publications

Braddock, SW. 1996. Straight Talk About Breast Cancer: From Diagnosis to Recovery: A Guide for the Entire Family.

Carney KL. 1998. What is Cancer Anyway? Explaining Cancer to Children of All Ages.

Davies K, White M. 1996. Breakthrough: The Race To Find The Breast Cancer Gene. A history of the discovery of the BRCA1 gene, including information on current treatments and future research directions.

DeGregorio, MW, Wiebe VJ. 1999. Tamoxifen and Breast Cancer.

Hapham WH. 1997. When a Parent Has Cancer: A Guide to Caring for Your Children.

Hapham WH. 2001. The Hope Tree: Kids Talk About Breast Cancer.

Harris JR, Hellman S, Henderson IC, Kinne DW. 1991. Breast Diseases.

Kahane, DH. 1995. No Less a Woman: Femininity, Sexuality & Breast Cancer.

Kalter S. 1987. Looking Up: The Complete Guide to Looking and Feeling Good for the Recovering Cancer Patient. Provides tips (with photos) on hair care, wigs, makeup, and exercise. (Out of print; check your local library to find a copy.)

Kohlenberg S. 1993. Sammy's Mommy Has Cancer.

Appendix

Landay D. 1998. Be Prepared: The Complete Financial, Legal, and Practical Guide for Living with a Life-Challenging Condition.

Link J. 1998. The Breast Cancer Survival Manual: A Step-By-Step Guide for the Woman With Newly Diagnosed Cancer.

Love, Susan M. 2000. Dr. Susan Love's Breast Book.

Marchant D. 1997. Breast Disease.

Moch SD, Graubard, A. 1996. Breast Cancer: Twenty Women's Stories: Becoming More Alive Through the Experience. (Out of print; check your local library.)

Phillips, RH, Goldstein P. 1998. Coping with Breast Cancer: A Practical Guide to Understanding, Treating, and Living with Breast Cancer.

Porter, ME (Editor), et al. 1997. Hope Is Contagious: The Breast Cancer Treatment Survival Handbook.

Porter, Margit Esser (Editor), et al. 2000. Hope Lives! The After Breast Cancer Treatment Survival Handbook (sequal to Hope Is Contagious)

Stumm, D. 1995. Recovering from Breast Surgery: Exercises to Strengthen Your Body and Relieve Pain.

Swirsky, J. et al. 1998. Coping With Lymphedema: Practical Guide to Understanding, Treating, and Living With Lymphedema

Torrey L. 1999. Michael's Mommy Has Breast Cancer.

Walker, LJ. 2000. Thanks for the Mammogram!: Fighting Cancer With Faith, Hope, and a Healthy Dose of Laughter.

Weiss, M. 1998. Living Beyond Breast Cancer: A Survivor's Guide for When Treatment Ends and The Rest of Your Life Begins.

Zuckweiler, R. 1998. Living in the Postmastectomy Body: Learning to Live in and Love Your Body Again.

Selected References

Sexuality and Intimacy

Fitzpatrick T, Johnson R, Polano M, Suurmond D, Wolff K. *Color Atlas and Synopsis of Clinical Dermatology* Second edition, p. 176.

Ganz P, Desmond K, Belin T, Meyerwitz B, Rowland J. *Predictors of Sexual Health in Women After a Breast Cancer Diagnosis.* Journal of Clinical Oncology 1999; 17(8):2371–2380.

Gaston M, Porter G. *Prime Time: The African American Woman's Complete Guide to Midlife Health and Wellness.*

Hodern A. *Intimacy and Sexuality for the Woman with Breast Cancer.* Cancer Nursing 2000;23(3):230–235.

Kornblith A, Ligibel J. *Psychosocial and Sexual Functioning of Survivors of Breast Cancer.* Seminars in Oncology 30(6):799–813.

Rogers M, Kristjanson L. *The Impact on Sexual Functioning of Chemotherapy-Induced Menopause in Women with Breast Cancer.* Cancer Nursing 2002;25:67–63.

Schover L. SPIRIT - *Sisters Peer Counseling in Reproductive Issues After Treatment Workbook.* A research partnership between the University of Texas M.D. Anderson Cancer Center and Sisters Network®, Inc.

Stead M. *Sexual Dysfunction After Treatment for Gynecologic and Breast Malignancies.* Current Opinion in Obstetrics and Gynecology 15:57–61.

Wilmoth M, Sanders L. *Accept Me for Myself: African American Women's Issues After Breast Cancer.* Oncology Nursing 2001;28(5):875–879.

Breast Cancer Treatment and Fertility

Brzezinski A, Peretz T, Mor-Yosef, Schenker JG. *Ovarian Stimulation and Breast Cancer: Is There a Link?* Gynecol Oncol. 1994 Mar; 52(3):292–5.

Dow KH, Kuhn D. Online exclusive: *Fertility Options in Young Breast Cancer Survivors: A review of the Literature.* Oncol Nurs Forum. 31(3):E46–53.

Friedlander M, Thewes B. *Counting the Costs of Treatment: The reproductive and Gynecological Consequences of Adjuvant Therapy in Young Women with Breast Cancer.* Intern Med J. 2003 (Aug; 33(8):372–9.

Meirow D. *Reproduction Post-chemotherapy in Young Cancer Patients.* Mol Cell Endocrinol. 2000 Nov 27; 169(1–2):123–31.

Weiss HA, Troisi R, Rossing MA, Brogan D, Coates RJ, Gammon MD, Potischman N, Swanson CA, Brinton LA. *Fertility Problems and Breast Cancer Risk in Young Women: A Case-Control Study in the United States.* Cancer Causes Control. 1988 May; 9(3):331–9.

Breast Cancer and Pregnancy

Ibrahim EM, Ezzat AA, Baloush A, Hussain ZH, Mohammed GH. *Pregnancy-Associated Breast Cancer: A Case-Control Study in a Young Population with a High-Fertility Rate.* Med Oncol. 2000 Nov;17(4):293–3000.

Partridge, Ann H. Lesnikoski, Beth-Ann, Burstein, Harold J. *Treatment of Breast Cancer During Pregnancy.* 3(4):423–428.

WEBSITES

WWW.GETBCFACTS.COM
WWW.BCRESOURCE.ORG
WWW.BREASTCANCER.COM
WWW.BREASTCANCER.ORG
WWW.CANCER.GOV
WWW.FERTILEHOPE.ORG
WWW.LIVESTRONG.ORG
WWW.SEXUALHEALTH.COM
WWW.XANDRIA.COM

Glossary

acupuncture: a Chinese therapy involving the use of thin needles inserted into specific locations in the skin

acute lymphedema: a temporary condition that lasts less than 6 months in which the skin indents when touched and stays indented, but remains soft to the touch

acute pain: severe, short-term pain

acute-onset nausea and vomiting: usually occur a few minutes to several hours after the chemotherapy is given

adenosis: an enlargement of breast lobules

adjuncts: drugs that complement the chemotherapy regimen

adjuvant therapy: treatment given after the primary treatment to increase the chances of a cure, and treatment to prevent the cancer from recurring

adrenaline: a hormone triggered by an important or stressful event that prepares the body for "fight or flight" reactions

advance directives: legal documents that allow people to express their decisions regarding what they do and don't want to have done during their last weeks or months in case they become unable to communicate effectively

alternative therapy: medicines used in lieu of standard medical therapies

anaplastic: cells that lose the distinguishing characteristics of original tissue

anemia: low counts of red blood cells

anticipatory nausea and vomiting: learned from previous experiences with vomiting; anticipating that nausea and vomiting will occur as it did previously triggers the actual reflex

antiemetics: antinausea medications

antihormones: drugs that block hormones before they can bind to the receptors in a tumor

areola: the dark area around the nipple

aromatase inhibitors: drugs that suppress the body's production of estrogen by reducing production of the enzyme aromatase

atypical hyperplasia: a noncancerous breast disease characterized by a growth of abnormal cells within the breast duct or lobules; can signal an increased risk of developing cancer

axillary lymph node dissection: removal of lymph nodes in the armpit during the initial surgery; the nodes are then examined by a pathologist to determine if cancerous cells are present

benign: not cancerous

bilateral: both sides

biopsy: a procedure in which cells are collected for microscopic examination

bone scan: an X-ray that looks for signs of metastasis

brachytherapy: a form of internal radiation therapy

breakthrough vomiting: occurs despite treatment to prevent it and requires additional therapy

breast mass: an abnormal collection of tissue within the breast, which may be benign or malignant; a biopsy is usually necessary to distinguish benign from malignant masses

breast-reduction surgery: removes not only fat, but breast tissue as well, to make the contralateral breast match the breast that has been surgically altered

breast-reconstruction surgery: surgery done during or after mastectomy to restore the shape of the original breast; see also latissimus dorsi re-construction, transverse rectus abdominus muscle (TRAM) flap, and free-flap construction

calcifications: tiny mineral deposits in the breast tissue

cancer: a hard lump that may or may not be tender

carcinomas: cancers that form in the surface cells of different tissues

cell proliferation: rapid growth and reproduction of cells

cells: basic elements of tissues; the appearance and composition of individual cells are unique to the tissue they compose

chemotherapy: the use of chemical agents (drugs) to systemically treat cancer

chronic lymphedema: lymphedema that lasts for longer than 6 months

chronic pain: pain that is present for long periods of time, though not always at the same level of intensity

clinical trial: a study of a drug or treatment with a large group of people testing the treatment

colon cancer: cancer beginning in the colon

complementary therapy: medicines used in conjunction with standard therapies

computerized thermal imaging: analyzes temperature values to measure minute changes in physiological and metabolic activity

contralateral: opposite

core needle biopsy: incorporating a large needle to remove a small cylinder of tissue from the lump for analysis

cyclical: breast tenderness that varies over the menstrual cycle

cyst: a noncancerous, fluid-filled sac that feels like a soft lump or a tender spot

cytotoxic: the ability to kill fast-growing cells, both cancerous and noncancerous, by preventing them from dividing

DCIS: *See* ductal carcinoma in situ

deconditioning: fatigue, weakness, and dizziness caused by spending too much time at rest and asleep

delayed-onset vomiting: develops more than 24 hours after chemotherapy is given

dosimetrist: works with the oncologist and the radiation physicist to calculate the amount of radiation to be delivered

drains: consist of plastic tubing and suction bottles; the tube runs from under the incision to a bottle outside your body.

ductal carcinoma: cancer beginning in the lining of the ducts

ductal carcinoma in situ: a noninvasive cancer in which abnormal cells are found only in the lining of the milk duct of the breast

ducts: the passages within the breast that bring milk from the lobules to the nipple

durable power of attorney: allows a specific family member to legally make all your decisions, personal and financial, for you in case you become incapacitated

endocrine therapy: *see* hormonal therapy.

endometrium: uterine lining

epithelial: cells on the surface of a tissue

epithelial hyperplasia: a disease in which the cells lining the ducts or the lobules proliferate

estrogen: female hormone related to childbearing

estrogen-receptor downregulator: drug that attacks a tumor's estrogen receptors, damaging them so that they are unable to bind to estrogen

estrogen-receptor positive cancer: cancer that grows more rapidly with exposure to the hormone estrogen

external radiation therapy: the X-rays come from radioactive material outside the body and are directed at the breast by a machine

fibroadenoma: a smooth, rubbery, or hard lump that moves easily within the breast tissue

fibrocystic breast changes: lumpiness, tenderness, or pain at certain times of the month

fibrosis: thickening of fibrous tissue into a solid mass

field: the treatment site

fine needle aspiration biopsy: uses a very thin needle to collect fluid or cells directly from the mass for evaluation

food pyramid: a guideline developed by the USDA showing appropriate quantities of different food groups for balanced nutrition

free-flap construction: a breast reconstruction technique in which part

251

of the skin and fat from the buttocks is removed and grafted onto the mastectomy site

Gene amplification: a genetic mutation that results in multiple copies of a gene

guided imagery: a mind-body technique in which the patient visualizes and meditates upon images that encourage a positive immune response

gynecologist: a specialist in women's health

health care proxy: permits a designated person to make decisions regarding your medical treatment when you are unable to do so

HER2 overexpression: a genetic feature of some cancers in which a receptor for human epidermal growth factor receptor 2 (HER2) protein, which encourages cell growth, occurs excessively due to an alteration in the HER2 gene

histologic grade: describes how slow or fast the cancer is growing and progressing from stage to stage

hormonal therapy: treatment that blocks the effects of hormones upon cancers that depend on hormones to grow (also referred to as endocrine therapy)

hormone replacement therapy: administration of artificial estrogen and progesterone to alleviate the symptoms of menopause and to prevent health problems experienced by postmenopausal women, particularly osteoporosis

hypercalcemia: accelerated loss of calcium in the bones, leading to elevated levels of the mineral in the

bloodstream with symptoms such as nausea and confusion

hyperfractionated radiation therapy: the daily dose of radiation is given in smaller increments separated by 4 to 6 hours

hypnosis: a state of high concentration just on the edge of sleeping and wakefulness

incidence: the number of times a disease occurs within a population of people

incision biopsy: involves surgical removal of the entire mass for evaluation

inflammatory breast cancer: a rare, but aggressive, type of breast cancer characterized by symptoms resembling a skin infection or rash

informed consent: a process by which patients participating in a clinical study are provided with all available information regarding the experimental treatment prior to consenting to receive that treatment

intraductal carcinoma: *See* ductal carcinoma in situ

intramammary lymph nodes: normal lymph structures within the breasts

intraoperative radiation: a dose of radiation is given directly to the tumor site immediately after the surgery to remove the tumor

invasive cancer: cancer that breaks through normal breast tissue barriers and invades surrounding areas

latissimus dorsi reconstruction: the latissimus dorsi muscle (muscle on the back, below the shoulder) is used in creating a new breast following mastectomy; *see* breast reconstruction

living will: outlines what care you want in the event you become unable to communicate due to coma or heavy sedation

lobes: collections of lobules within the breast

lobular carcinoma: cancer formed in the lobules

lobular carcinoma in situ: abnormal cells are found in the lining of the milk lobule

lobules: individual glands within the lobes that secrete milk

lumpectomy: only the tumor and a small section of normal breast tissue are removed from the breast, leaving the breast virtually intact

lymph: fluid carried through the body by the lymphatic system, composed primarily of white blood cells and diluted plasma

lymph nodes: tissues in the lymphatic system that filter lymph fluid and help the immune system fight disease

lymphatic system: a collection of vessels with the principal functions of transporting digested fat from the intestine to the bloodstream, removing and destroying toxins from tissues, and resisting the spread of disease throughout the body

lymphedema: a condition in which lymph fluid collects in tissues following removal of, or damage to, lymph nodes during surgery, causing the limb or area of the body affected to swell; *see also* acute lymphedema and chronic lymphedema

macrocalcifications: large calcium deposits in the breast that appear on mammograms as spots within the breast tissue

malignant: cancerous; growing rapidly and out of control

mammogram/mammography: an X-ray examination of the breast

mastectomy/lumpectomy: involves surgical removal of the cancerous tissue and a certain amount of the surrounding tissue, sometimes including nodes from the nearby lymph system

medical oncologist: *see* oncologist

meditation: a mental technique that clears the mind and relaxes the body through concentration

menarche: start of menstruation

menopause: end of menstrual periods

metastasis, metastasize: the spread of cancer

microcalcifications: very small calcium deposits that appear on mammograms as tiny flecks

modified radical mastectomy: the surgeon removes the breast, some lymph nodes under the arm, and the lining over the chest muscles

mortality: the statistical calculation of death rates due to a specific disease or cause within a population

mutated: altered

mutation: a gene with a mistake or alteration

neoadjuvant therapy: adjuvant therapy that is started before the primary treatment

non-breast-origin pain: pain in the chest wall or ribs under the breast

noncyclical: constant pain in one spot that does not alter during the monthly menstrual cycle

noninvasive cancer: cancer confined to its tissue point of origin and not found in surrounding tissues

nonsteroidal anti-inflammatory drugs (NSAIDs): a class of pain medications, often sold over the counter, that includes ibuprofen and similar common pain killers

nutritionist: a health professional with specialized training in nutrition who can offer help with choices about the foods you eat

oncologist: a cancer specialist who helps determine treatment choices

opioids: medicines derived from morphine and similar chemicals

osteolytic lesions: small holes in the bones

osteoporosis: loss of bone density

ovarian cancer: cancer beginning in the ovaries, sometimes genetically related to breast cancer

Paget's disease: a rare cancer that begins in the milk ducts of the nipple

palliative care: care to relieve the symptoms of cancer and to keep the best quality of life for as long as possible without seeking to cure the cancer

palpation: carefully feeling the lump and the tissue around it

partial mastectomy: the surgeon removes the tumor, some of the normal breast tissue around it, and the lining over the chest muscles below the tumor

pathologist: a specialist trained to distinguish normal from abnormal cells

persistent pain: pain that is present for long periods of time, though not always at the same level of intensity

phases: a series of steps followed in clinical trials

phytoestrogens: natural, estrogen-like compounds in plant foods

placebos: sugar pills

plastic surgeon: a surgical specialist who will perform any reconstruction procedures that might be required

platelets: components of blood that assist in clotting and wound healing

port: the treatment site

primary care doctor: regular physician who gives check-ups

primary prevention: any treatment method or lifestyle change that directly prevents cancer cells from forming, growing, or multiplying

progesterone-receptor positive cancer: cancer that grows more rapidly with exposure to the hormone progesterone

progestin: a synthetic form of progesterone often used in birth control pills and hormone replacement therapy

prognosis: an estimation of the likely outcome of an illness based upon the patient's current status and the available treatments

prophylactic mastectomy: removal of a healthy breast in high-risk women to prevent the possible development of cancer at a later time

protocols: the research plan for how the drug is given and to whom it is given

radiologist: a physician specializing in treatment of disease using radiation therapy

radiation oncologist: a cancer specialist who determines the amount of radiotherapy required

radiation nurse: coordinates radiation therapy and patient care, helps patients learn about treatment, and assists in management of side effects

radiation physicist: makes sure that the equipment is working properly and that the machines deliver the right dose of radiation

radiation therapist: positions patients for radiation treatments and runs the equipment that delivers the radiation

radiation therapy: use of high-energy X-rays to kill cancer cells and shrink tumors

radical mastectomy (also called Halsted radical mastectomy): removal of both of the two chest muscles, as well as the breast and lymph nodes

radiofrequency ablation: use of high-frequency alternating current to create frictional heat within the tumor to "burn" the tumor cells to death without the need to actually cut open the breast and remove them

radiosurgery ablation: uses robotic devices and imaging software to target specific areas with high-energy beams of radiation

recurrent cancer: the disease has come back in spite of the initial treatment

red blood cells: cells in the blood with the primary function of carrying oxygen to tissues

risk factors: any factors that contribute to an increased possibility of getting cancer

sarcomas: cancers that form in connective tissues

secondary prevention: treatments or lifestyle changes that limit a person's exposure to cancer risk factors, but don't directly prevent the formation of cancer

segmental mastectomy: removal of tumor, some of the normal breast tissue around it, and the lining over the chest muscles below the tumor

selective estrogen receptor modulators (SERMs): drugs that bind to the estrogen receptor, blocking estrogen from binding to tumor cells

sentinel node biopsy: addition of dye during breast surgery to help locate the first lymph node attached to the cancerous zone; the node is then removed to prevent spread of cancer and biopsied to determine whether cancerous cells are present

simulation: a practice treatment that allows the team to determine exactly where they want the radioactive beams to be applied

stage: a numerical determination of how far the cancer has progressed

stereotactic: computer-guided imaging

surgical biopsy: removes a portion of the mass for further evaluation

surgical oncologist: a specialist trained in surgical removal of cancerous tumors

targeted therapy: treatment that targets specific molecules involved in carcinogenesis or tumor growth

telangiectasias: small, red areas appear on the skin, caused by dilation in blood vessels of the skin

total (simple) mastectomy: the surgeon removes the whole breast but does not remove lymph nodes

transverse rectus abdominus muscle (TRAM) flap: a muscle from the abdomen, along with skin and fat, is transferred to the mastectomy site and shaped like a breast. *See also* breast reconstruction

tumor: mass or lump of extra tissue

ultrasonography: uses sound waves to determine whether a lump is solid or filled with fluid

unilateral: one side

unsealed internal radiation therapy: a technique in which a solution of radioactive substances is injected directly into the bloodstream

uterine cancer: cancer beginning in the uterus; sometimes related genetically to breast cancer

white blood cells: cells in the blood with the primary function of combating infection

xenoestrogens: chemical compounds, usually industrial or pesticidal, that have similar effects in the body as estrogen

Index

Index